DEMONSTRATING YOUR COMPETENCE IN REPRODUCTIVE HEALTH – A GUIDE FOR HOSPITAL DOCTORS, THEIR TRAINERS AND PRACTITIONERS WITH A SPECIAL INTEREST

Julian Jenkins

Stephen Keay

Gill Wakley

Ruth Chambers

Forewords by
William Dunlop
and
Steve Field

RADCLIFFE PUBLISHING
Oxford ● Seattle

Radcliffe Publishing Ltd
18 Marcham Road
Abingdon
Oxon OX14 1AA
United Kingdom

www.radcliffe-oxford.com
Electronic catalogue and worldwide online ordering facility.

© 2005 Julian Jenkins, Stephen Keay, Gill Wakley and Ruth Chambers

British Library Cataloguing in Publication Data

A catalogue record for this book is available from the British Library.

ISBN 1 85775 620 7

Typeset by Advance Typesetting Ltd, Oxford
Printed and bound by T J International, Padstow, Cornwall

Contents

Foreword

Times are changing. Until recently doctors were expected to keep up to date in their practice but did not need to demonstrate continuing competence. They faced sanctions only if their management of patients resulted in problems serious enough to be brought to the attention of the General Medical Council or the civil or criminal courts. Relatively few cases did. Doctors and their patients assumed that all was well and that British doctors could be trusted to deliver up-to-date treatment of high quality.

During the last years of the 20th century, however, these assumptions were severely challenged by a series of high-profile cases that clearly demonstrated that individual doctors and teams, many of whom were respected by their patients, could have serious deficiencies in their practice leading to inappropriate, inadequate or even dangerous management. There was clearly need for change. It would henceforth be necessary for doctors to be able to demonstrate objectively and transparently that they were maintaining a standard of clinical practice that was deemed appropriate by their peers and acceptable by the public.

At the time of writing, the precise details of how this is to be achieved remain somewhat unclear. The General Medical Council has approved the principle that registered medical practitioners should be licensed to practise only if they can demonstrate that they have undergone an approved revalidation process. This process is currently under review but it is clear that it will be essential for doctors to keep records showing that they have audited aspects of their practice and that it meets appropriate standards. This will be a daunting prospect for many.

Those doctors whose practice involves obstetrics and gynaecology are, however, better placed than most to implement the process. The Royal College of Obstetricians and Gynaecologists (RCOG) was the first to develop a coherent programme of Continuing Professional Development and, building on this foundation, to set out guidelines for the revalidation of specialists in the field. Simultaneously other groups within the College were developing evidence-based guidelines for the management of common clinical problems in both obstetrics and gynaecology. Care was taken to involve the relevant specialist societies in the development of the guidelines and to ensure that the views of non-specialists were also taken into consideration. The guidelines proved to be both popular and effective. The methodology was well established when the National Institute for Clinical Excellence (NICE) was established and it was a relatively straightforward matter to transform RCOG guidelines into NICE guidelines. In consequence, there now exists a well-respected, comprehensively reviewed database defining the delivery of acceptable contemporary clinical care in obstetrics and gynaecology. This provides an ideal resource for doctors who need to evaluate their personal practice.

This excellent book takes the process one stage further. It sets out a methodology whereby a doctor whose practice involves reproductive health (whether as a specialist or as a general practitioner with a special interest) can document the audit and improvement of professional skills. The technique is innovative, practical and valuable. It has the potential to be applied not only in the field of obstetrics and gynaecology, but to many other clinical disciplines. I look forward eagerly to further publications in this series.

Professor William Dunlop CBE
Former President
Royal College of Obstetricians and Gynaecologists
December 2004

Foreword

I am delighted to write the foreword for this book whose arrival is timely given the General Medical Council's revalidation reforms which take effect from April 2005. Inevitably, at times of change there will be anxiety about what these changes mean and how individual doctors can satisfy the new requirements to continue to practise in the UK.

I am sure that this book will help to alleviate those anxieties by removing the 'fear of the unknown' through a series of concise chapters covering the crucial clinical areas in reproductive healthcare. I commend the excellent practical advice on how to accumulate revalidation data by using practical examples based on cycles of evidence.

Revalidation will change the emphasis of regulation away from the qualifications of MRCOG or DRCOG towards regular assessment of the doctor's competence to practise. It will be incumbent upon us as individual doctors, whether in training or in substantive posts in primary or secondary care, to reflect on our work and to demonstrate our competence to practise. For training grades (SHOs, SpRs), secondary care career grades (consultants and staff grade doctors in Obstetrics & Gynaecology) and general practitioners with a special interest (GPwSI) in reproductive health, this book will be an invaluable aid to negotiating this transition of having to formally demonstrate competence. Increasing numbers of non-UK medically qualified doctors are practising in the UK (accounting for 30% of our own Deanery in the West Midlands) and this publication will provide them with clear guidance on the sort of information that should be collected to support their revalidation.

I envisage that many of us involved in reproductive health will refer to this book time and again, particularly as our licence renewal draws near, to adapt the cycles of evidence to our own needs. *Demonstrating your Competence in Reproductive Health* is an excellent contribution that will help doctors immensely in their preparation for the requirements of revalidation in all aspects of reproductive health.

Professor Steve Field
Regional Postgraduate Dean
West Midlands
December 2004

Preface

From April 2005 the General Medical Council requires doctors to collect and keep the information that will show that they should continue to hold a licence to practise as doctors. The onus will be on individual doctors to show that they are up to date and fit to practise medicine throughout their careers. It will be doctors who decide for themselves the nature of the information they collect and retain that best reflects their roles and responsibilities in their everyday work.

This book is one of a series that will guide you as a doctor though the process, giving you examples and ideas as to how to document your learning, competence, performance or standards of service delivery. Chapter 1 explains the link between your personal development plans, local appraisal and the revalidation of your medical registration. Learning and service improvements that are integral to your personal development plan are central to the evidence you include in your appraisal and revalidation portfolio.

The stages of the evidence cycle that we suggest are built upon the underpinning publication: Chambers R, Wakley G, Field S and Ellis S (2002) *Appraisal for the Apprehensive*. Radcliffe Medical Press, Oxford.

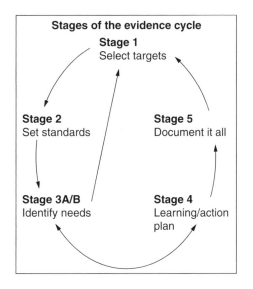

Stages of the evidence cycle

Stage 1
Select targets

Stage 2
Set standards

Stage 5
Document it all

Stage 3A/B
Identify needs

Stage 4
Learning/action plan

Stage 1 is about setting targets or aspirations for good practice. Many of the aspirations we suggest are taken from *Good Medical Practice*[1] or its sister publications, *Revalidation in Obstetrics and Gynaecology Criteria, Standards and Evidence*[2] and *Good Medical Practice for General Practitioners.*[3] Stage 2 encourages you as a doctor to set standards for the outcomes of what you plan to learn more about, or outcomes relating to you providing a good service in your practice.

Chapters 1 to 4 describe a variety of methods to help you to address Stage 3 of the cycle of evidence, to find out what it is you need to learn about or what gaps there are in the way you deliver care as an individual doctor or as a team. These chapters include a wide variety of methods doctors might use in their everyday work to identify and document these needs. One of the drivers for the introduction of appraisal and revalidation has been to reassure the public and others of doctors' continuing fitness to practise. So it makes sense that we have emphasised the importance of obtaining feedback from patients in relation to identifying your learning and service development needs. These chapters also look at methods of learning and teaching and ways in which you might meet your learning needs.

Best practice in addressing the giving of informed consent by patients, maintaining confidentiality of patient information and organising responsive complaints processes are all common components of good quality healthcare. Confidentiality is also important during training activities.

The rest of the book consists of six clinically based chapters that span key topics in reproductive health. The first part of each chapter covers key issues that are likely to crop up in typical consultations for each clinical field. The second part of each chapter gives examples of cycles of evidence.

Overall, you will probably want to choose three or four cycles of evidence each year. You might like this way of learning and service development so much that you build up a bigger bank of evidence, taking one cycle from each chapter in the same year. Whatever your approach, you will want to keep your cycles of evidence as short and simple as possible, so that the documentation itself is a by-product of the learning and action plans you undertake to improve the service you provide, and does not dominate your time and effort at work.

Other books in the series are based on the same format of the five stages in the cycle of evidence. Book 1 helps doctors and other health professionals to demonstrate that they are competent teachers or trainers, and other books give key information for general practitioners or nurses wishing to demonstrate their competence in a variety of clinical subjects.

This approach and style of learning will take a bit of getting used to for doctors. Until now, they have not had to prove that they are fit to practise unless the General Medical Council has investigated them for a significant reason such as a complaint or error. Until recently, most doctors did not evaluate what they learnt or whether they applied it in practice. They did not protect time for learning and reflection among their everyday responsibilities, or target their time and effort on priority topics. Times are changing, and with the introduction of personal development plans and appraisal, doctors are realising that they must take a more professional approach to learning and document their standards of competence, performance and service delivery. This book helps them to do just that.

Please note that resources to support this book are provided at http://health.mattersonline.net.

References

1   General Medical Council (2001) *Good Medical Practice*. General Medical Council, London.

2   Royal College of Obstetricians and Gynaecologists (2002) *Revalidation in Obstetrics and Gynaecology Criteria, Standards and Evidence*. Royal College of Obstetricians and Gynaecologists Press, London.

3   Royal College of General Practitioners/General Practitioners Committee (2002) *Good Medical Practice for General Practitioners*. Royal College of General Practitioners, London.

About the authors

Julian Jenkins has had a longstanding involvement in postgraduate education and many initiatives including novel applications of learning technology. He is a consultant senior lecturer and the clinical director of the Centre for Reproductive Medicine at the University of Bristol (www.ReproMED.co.uk). He is the course director of an innovative MSc course in reproduction and development delivered principally over the internet (www.ReD-MSc.org.uk) and the chairman of the obstetrics and gynaecology education subcommittee for the South West Region (www.swot.org.uk). For many years, he has been involved with the development of evidence-based medicine as a member of the Royal College of Obstetricians and Gynaecologists' Guidelines and Audit Committee and the Menstrual Disorder and Infertility Panel of the Cochrane Collaboration.

Stephen Keay is a consultant senior lecturer in obstetrics and gynaecology in the Department of Biological Sciences, University of Warwick and University Hospitals Coventry and Warwickshire NHS Trust. He is involved in the teaching of Warwick Medical School students and is an external reviewer for the undergraduate programme at the University of Bristol. His main clinical interests are in infertility and reproductive endocrinology. He is a member of the Menstrual Disorder and Infertility Panel of the Cochrane Collaboration.

Gill Wakley started in general practice but transferred to community medicine shortly afterwards and then into public health. A desire for increased contact with patients caused a move back into general practice. She has been heavily involved in learning and teaching throughout her career. She was in a training general practice, became an instructing doctor and a regional assessor in family planning, and was, until recently, a senior clinical lecturer with the Primary Care Department at Keele University. Like Ruth, she has run all types of educational initiatives and activities. A visiting professor at Staffordshire University, she now works as a freelance GP, writer and lecturer.

Ruth Chambers has been a GP for more than 20 years and is currently the head of the Stoke-on-Trent Teaching Primary Care Trust programme and clinical dean at Staffordshire University. Ruth has worked with the Royal College of General Practitioners to enable GPs to gather evidence about their learning and standards of practice whilst striving to be excellent GPs. Ruth has co-authored a series of books with Gill designed to help readers draw up their own personal development plans or workplace learning plans around key clinical topics.

1

Making the link: personal development plans, appraisal and revalidation

The nexus of personal development plans, appraisal and revalidation

Learning involves many steps. It includes the acquisition of information, its retention, the ability to retrieve the information when needed and how to use that information for best practice. Demonstrating your learning involves being able to show the steps you have taken. Learning should be lifelong and encompass continuing professional development.

Professional training including continuing professional development (CPD) takes time. Whatever your position, it makes sense to utilise the time spent by overlapping learning to meet your personal and professional needs, with that required for the performance of your role in the health service.

While in training you may have clear objectives leading towards a formal qualification or as part of your structured training programme. Having achieved a substantive appointment, it may be less clear how to plan your learning. You could draw up a personal development plan (PDP) that is agreed with your local CPD or college tutor. Some doctors have constructed their PDP in a systematic way and identified the priorities within it, or gathered evidence to demonstrate that what they learnt about was subsequently applied in practice. Tutors do not have a uniform approach to the style and relevance of a doctor's PDP. Some are content that a plan has been drawn up, while others encourage the doctor to develop a systematic approach to identifying and addressing their learning and service needs, in order of importance or urgency.[1]

The new emphasis on doctors' accountability to the public has given the PDP a higher profile and shown that the PDP may be used in other ways. The medical education establishment and NHS management argue about the balance between its alternative uses. The educationalists view a personal development plan as a tool to encourage doctors to plan their own learning activities. The management view is of a tool allowing quality assurance of the doctor's performance. Doctors, striving to improve the quality of the care that they deliver to patients, want to use a personal development plan to guide them on their way, perhaps towards postgraduate awards of universities or the quality awards of the Royal Colleges. These quality awards are built around the standards of excellence to which a doctor should aspire, as described in the publication, *Good Medical Practice*.[2–4]

Your personal development plan

Your PDP will be an integral part of your future appraisal and revalidation portfolio to demonstrate your fitness to practise as a doctor.
   Your initial plan should:

- identify your gaps or weaknesses in knowledge, skills or attitudes
- specify topics for learning as a result of changes: in your role, responsibilities, the organisation in which you work
- link into the learning needs of others in your workplace or team of colleagues
- tie in with the service development priorities of your practice, the primary care organisation (PCO) or the NHS as a whole
- describe how you identified your learning needs
- set your learning needs and associated goals in order of importance and urgency
- justify your selection of learning goals
- describe how you will achieve your goals and over what time period
- describe how you will evaluate learning outcomes.

Each year you will continue or revise your PDP. It should demonstrate how you carried out your learning and evaluation plans, show that you have learnt what you set out to do (or why it was modified) and how you applied your new learning in practice. In addition, you will find that you have new priorities and fresh learning needs as circumstances change.
   The main task is to capture what you have learnt, in a way that suits you. Then you can look back at what you have done and:

- reflect on it later, to decide to learn more, or to make changes as a result, and identify further needs
- demonstrate to others that you are fit to practise or work through:
  - what you have done
  - what you have learnt
  - what changes you have made as a result
  - the standards of work you have achieved and are maintaining
  - how you monitor your performance at work

- use it to show how your personal learning fits in with the requirements of your practice or the NHS, and other people's personal and professional development plans.

Organise all the evidence of your learning into a CPD portfolio of some sort. It is up to you how you keep this record of your learning. Examples are:

- *an ongoing learning journal* in which you draw up and describe your plan, record how you determined your needs and prioritised them, report why you attended particular educational meetings or courses and what you got out of them as well as the continuing cycle of review, making changes and evaluating them
- *an A4 file* with lots of plastic sleeves into which you build up a systematic record of your educational activities in line with your plan
- *a box*: chuck in everything to do with your learning plan as you do it and sort it out into a sensible order every few months with a good review once a year.

The context of appraisal and revalidation

Appraisal and revalidation are based on the same sources of information – presented in the same structure as the headings set out in the General Medical Council (GMC) guidance in *Good Medical Practice*.[4] The two processes perform different functions. Whereas revalidation involves an assessment against a standard of fitness to practise medicine, appraisal is concerned with the doctor's professional development within his or her working environment and the needs of the organisation for which the doctor works.

Appraisal is a formative and developmental process that is being introduced by the Departments of Health for all general practitioners (GPs) and hospital consultants working in the NHS across the UK. While the details of the appraisal system vary for consultants and GPs and for each of the countries, the educational principles remain the same. The aims of the appraisal system are to give doctors an opportunity to discuss and receive regular feedback on their previous and continuing performance and identify education and development needs.

The drive to introduce formal appraisals came initially as part of the programme to introduce clinical governance across the NHS as laid out in the 1998 consultation document *A First Class Service*.[5] Momentum was gained with the publication of *Supporting Doctors, Protecting Patients* (1999) in England which outlined a set of proposals to help prevent doctors from developing problems.[6] Appraisal was at the heart of the proposals as:

a positive process to give someone feedback on their performance, to chart their continuing progress and to identify development needs. It is a forward looking process essential for the developmental and educational planning needs of an individual. *Assessment* is the process of measuring progress against agreed criteria .... It is not the primary aim of appraisal to scrutinise doctors to see if they are performing poorly but rather to help them consolidate and improve on good performance aiming towards excellence.[5]

The document went on to suggest that appraisal should be made comprehensive and compulsory for doctors working in the NHS and form part of a future revalidation system.

In addition, appraisal should also address other areas of particular importance to the individual doctor. A standardised approach has been developed which utilises approved documentation. This should ensure that information from a variety of NHS employers is recorded consistently. The format of the paperwork is slightly different for consultants and GPs.

Appraisal must be a positive, formative and developmental process to support high quality patient care and improve clinical standards. Appraisal is different from, but linked to, revalidation.[6] Revalidation is the process whereby doctors will be regularly required to demonstrate that they are fit to practise. Appraisal feeds into this by contributing to the information that a doctor supplies for the revalidation process. Appraisal will provide a regular structured recording system for documenting progress towards revalidation and identifying needs as part of the doctor's PDP. Both the NHS appraisal and the revalidation structures are based on the same seven headings set out in the GMC's guidance *Good Medical Practice*.[4] The GMC provides guidance regarding the revalidation process, which will vary depending on the circumstances of individual doctors.[7] The GMC has explained that doctors not taking part in appraisal will be able to provide their own information for revalidation, providing this evidence meets the same criteria as in *Good Medical Practice*.[4]

Appraisal is, however, a two-way process. Not only time, but also resources will be needed to make appraisal systems successful. In addition, appraisal will identify issues that will require extra investment by the NHS in the educational and organisational infrastructure.

Appraisal and revalidation processes are being increasingly integrated. The PDP is a central part of the appraisal documentation, which will in turn be included in the portfolio of information available for revalidation. It seems that the evolution will continue so that revalidation is met by supporting the appraisal documentation with additional documents about clinical governance activity and CPD. These supporting documents will be a mix of subjective and objective information that will include doctors' self-assessment of their performance and other work-based assessment.

The revalidation and appraisal processes need to be quality assured to be able to demonstrate that they can protect the public from poor or under-performing doctors. Such quality assurance will relate to the appraisers, their training and support, as well as systems to examine the quality of evidence in the documentation relating to a doctor's performance and outcomes of their PDP. You should regard your PDP and supporting documentation as central to the way in which you can show, to anyone who requires you to do so, that your performance as a doctor is acceptable and that you are trying to improve, or striving for excellence.

Demonstrating the standards of your practice

The GMC sets out standards that must be met as part of the duties and responsibilities of doctors in the booklet *Good Medical Practice*.[4] Doctors must be able to meet these standards with a record of their own performance in their revalidation portfolio if they want to retain a licence to practise. The key headings of expected standards of practice are outlined in Box 1.1.

Box 1.1:   Key headings of expected standards of practice for doctors working in the UK

1 *Good professional practice.* This relates to clinical care, keeping records (including writing reports and keeping colleagues informed), access and availability, treatment in emergencies and making effective use of resources.
2 *Maintaining good medical practice.* This includes keeping up to date and maintaining your performance.
3 *Relationships with patients.* This encompasses providing information about your services, maintaining trust, avoiding discrimination and prejudice against patients, relating well to patients and apologising if things go wrong.
4 *Working with colleagues.* This relates to working with colleagues, working in teams, referring patients and accepting posts.
5 *Teaching and training, appraising and assessing.* You may be in a position to teach or train colleagues or students, and appraise or assess peers, employees or students.
6 *Probity* includes providing true information about your services, honesty in financial and commercial dealings, and providing references.
7 *Health* can include how you overcome or compensate for health problems in yourself, or help with or address health problems in other doctors.
8 *Research.* Conducting research in an ethical manner.
9 *Management.** The section on management concerns any responsibility doctors have for management outside their practice. Some doctors of various specialties are not required to consider management separately.

---

*Appraisal paperwork has been individualised for each college and separately for GPs working in England, Scotland, Wales and Northern Ireland.

The stages of the evidence cycle for demonstrating your standards of practice or competence and any necessary improvements are given in Figure 1.1. The stages of the evidence cycle are common to all the various areas of expertise considered in this book and will be followed in each chapter.

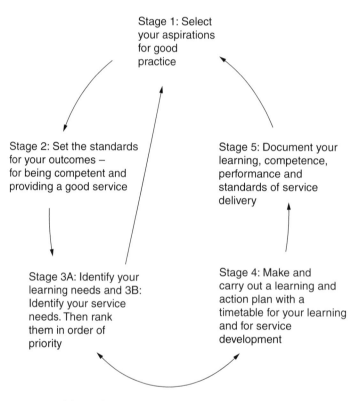

Figure 1.1: Stages of the evidence cycle.

Although the five stages are shown in sequence here, in practice you would expect to move backwards and forwards from stage to stage, because of new information or a modification of your earlier ideas. New information might accrue when research is published which affects your clinical behaviour or standards, or a critical incident or patient complaint might occur which causes you and others to think anew about your standards or the way that services are delivered. The arrows in Figure 1.1 show that you might reset your target or aspirations for good practice having undertaken exercises to identify what you need to learn or determine if there are gaps in service delivery.

We suggest that you demonstrate your competence in focused areas of your day-to-day work by completing several cycles of evidence drawn from a variety of clinical or other areas each year, with at least one cycle of evidence from each of the main headings of *Good Medical Practice* over a five-year cycle.[4] By demonstrating your standards of practice around the main sections of *Good Medical Practice*, you will document your competence and performance for your revalidation portfolio in the same format as that required for your appraisal paperwork.

As you start to collate information about this five-stage cycle, discuss any problems about the standards of care or services you are looking at, with colleagues, experts in this area, tutors, etc. You want to develop a wide range and depth of evidence so that you can show that you are competent in your day-to-day general work as well as for any special areas of expertise.

Professional competence is the first area of concern in *Good Medical Practice*.[4] You should be able to demonstrate that you can maintain a satisfactory standard of clinical care most of the time in your everyday work. Some of the time you will be brilliant, of course! Celebrate those moments. On other occasions, you or others will be critical of your performance and feel that you could have done much better. Reflect on those episodes to learn from them.

Stage 1: Select your aspirations for good practice

By adopting or adapting descriptions of what an 'excellent' doctor should be aiming for, you are defining the standards of practice for which all doctors should be aiming. The medical Royal Colleges have interpreted *Good Medical Practice* in various ways for the specialties of their own members.[4] *Revalidation in Obstetrics and Gynaecology Criteria, Standards and Evidence* sets standards that specialists would be expected to achieve most of the time.[2] Similarly *Good Medical Practice for General Practitioners* describes the standards of practice that should be achieved by 'excellent' or 'unacceptable' general practitioners.[3] Their definition of excellence is being 'consistently good'.[5]

Consistency is a critical factor in considering competence and performance. The documents that you collect in your evidence cycles must reflect consistency over time and in different circumstances, for example with various types of patients or your work at different times of day. This will show that you have not only performed well on one occasion or for one type of baseline assessment, but also sustained your performance over time and under different conditions.

Stage 2: Set the standards for your outcomes – for being competent and providing a good service

Outcomes might include:

- the way that learning is applied
- a learnt skill
- a protocol
- a strategy that is implemented
- meeting recommended standards.

The level at which you should be performing depends on your particular field of expertise. Some gynaecologists may have a very narrow focus but have high standards of expertise in that field. They might regard themselves as lacking competence in other fields and need to be selective in accepting the type of patient referred to them. Others may have a more general field of work and will aspire to be competent at a broad range of activities, while recognising the need to refer on when their limits of expertise are reached.

Other standards include using resources effectively and the record keeping that is an essential tool in clinical care. As a health professional, you need to be accessible and available so that you can provide your services, and make suitable arrangements for handing over care to others. You must provide care in an emergency.

You could incorporate into your standards or outcomes those components specified by universities at a national level as part of their Masters' Frameworks for their postgraduate awards. The Masters' Frameworks consist of eight components that shape the individual postgraduate award programme outcomes and the learning outcomes of the individual modules for the postgraduate awards. The eight components are shown in Box 1.2. You could set out your CPD work in the portfolio you are assembling for revalidation and your annual appraisals in this format. This would help you to document your professional development to date in a form that can be readily 'accredited for prior experiential learning' (APEL) by universities (contact your local universities if you want more information about this process). You might then be given credits for learning against an intended postgraduate award. It would save you from duplicating work as well as speeding your progress through the award.

Box 1.2:   The eight components of the Masters Frameworks for postgraduate awards

1   Analysis
2   Problem solving
3   Knowledge and understanding

4 Reflection
5 Communication
6 Learning
7 Application
8 Enquiry

If you have information or data about your work showing that it was substandard or that you were not competent, you might choose to exclude that from your portfolio. However, you will be able to show that you have learnt more by reviewing mistakes or negative episodes. It is better to include everything of relevance, then go on to demonstrate how you addressed the gaps in your performance and made sustained improvements. You will need to protect the confidentiality of patients and colleagues as necessary when you collect data. The GMC will be seeing the contents of your revalidation portfolio if your submission is one of those sampled. You will probably also submit or share the documentation for appraisal and maybe use it for reviews with colleagues or the trust.

Stage 3: Identify your learning and service needs in your work or trust and rank them in order of priority[1]

The type and depth of documentation you need to gather will encompass:

• the context in which you work
• your knowledge and skills in relation to any particular role or responsibility of your current post.

The extent of expertise you should possess will depend on your level of responsibility for a particular function or task. You may be personally responsible for that function or task, or you may contribute or delegate responsibility for it. Your learning needs should take into account your aspirations for the future too – personal or career development for you, or improvements in the way you deliver care.

Group and summarise your service development needs from the exercises you have carried out. Grade them according to the priority you set. You may put one at a higher priority because it fits in with service development needs established in the business plan of the trust or department, or put another lower because it does not fit in with other activities that your organisation has in their current development plan for the next 12 months. If you have identified a service development need by several different methods of assessment or with several different patient groups or clinical conditions, then it will have a higher priority than something only identified once. Notify the service development needs you have identified to those responsible for agreeing and implementing the development plans of the trust and/or department.

Look back at your aspirations and standards set out in Stages 1 and 2. Match your learning or service development needs with one or more of these standards, or others that you have set yourself.

Stage 4: Make and carry out a learning and action plan with a timetable for your personal and service development

If you have not identified any learning needs for yourself or the service as a whole, you should omit Stage 4 and tidy up the presentation of your evidence for inclusion in your portfolio as at the end of Stage 5.

Think about whether:

- you have defined your learning objectives – what you need to learn to be able to attain the standards and outcomes you have described in Stage 2
- you can justify spending time and effort on the topics you prioritised in Stage 3. Is the topic important enough to your work, the NHS as a whole or patient safety? Does the clinical or non-clinical event occur sufficiently often to warrant the time spent?
- the time and resources for learning about that topic or making the associated changes to service delivery are available. Check that you are not trying to do too much too quickly, or you will become discouraged
- learning about that topic will make a difference to the care you or others can provide for patients
- and how one topic fits in with other topics you have identified to learn more about. Have you achieved a good balance across your areas of work or between your personal aspirations and the basic requirements of the service?

Decide on what method of learning is most appropriate for your task or role or the standards you are expecting to attain or sustain. You may have already identified your preferred learning style – but read up on this elsewhere if you are unsure.[8] There are more ideas about how to learn in the following chapters.

Describe how you will carry out your learning tasks and what you will do by a specified time. State how your learning will be applied and how and when it will be evaluated. Build in some staging posts so that you do not suddenly get to the end of 12 months and discover that you have only done half of your plan.

Your action plan should also include your role in remedying any gaps in service delivery that you identified in Stage 3 that are within the remit of your responsibility.

Stage 5: Document your learning, competence, performance and standards of service delivery

You might choose to document that you have attained your defined outcomes by repeating the learning needs assessment that you started with. You could record your increased confidence and competence in dealing with situations that you previously avoided or performed inadequately.

You might incorporate your assessment of what has been gained in a study of another area that overlaps.

Preparing your portfolio[9-11]

Use your portfolio of evidence of what you have learnt and your standards of practice to:

- identify significant experiences to serve as important sources of learning
- reflect on the learning that arose from those experiences
- demonstrate learning in practice
- analyse and identify further learning needs and ways in which these needs can be met.

Your documentation might include all sorts of things, not just formal audits – although they make a good start. It might include reports of educational activities attended, statements of your roles and responsibilities, copies of publications you have read and critically appraised, and reports of your work. You could incorporate observations by others, evaluations of you observing other colleagues and how their practice differs from yours, descriptions of self-improvements, a video of typical activity, materials that demonstrate your skills to others, products of your input or learning – a new protocol for example. Box 1.3 gives a list of material you might include in your portfolio.

Box 1.3: Possible contents of a portfolio

Workload logs:

- gynaecology outpatient clinics
  - number of new cases in a year
  - number of follow-up cases in a year

- theatre lists
  - number of majors in a year
  - number of minors in a year
- deliveries
  - number of patients booked in a year
  - breakdown of outcomes

And:

- thank you letters from patients
- case descriptions
- patient satisfaction surveys
- audit or research surveys
- contributions to any local, regional, national or international professional bodies
- report of change or innovation
- publications and presentations
- records of critical incidents and learning points
- notes from formal teaching sessions with reference to clinical work or other evidence

Once you are preparing to submit the portfolio for a discussion with a colleague (for example, at an appraisal) or assessment (for example, for a university postgraduate award or revalidation), write a self-assessment of your previous action plan. You might integrate your self-assessment into your PDP to show what you have achieved and what gaps you have still to address. Decide where you are now and where you want to be in one, three or five years' time. Select items from your portfolio for inclusion for each part of the documentation – you might have one compartment of your portfolio per specialty topic or section heading from *Good Medical Practice*.[4]

Make sure all references are included and the documentation in your portfolio is as accurate and complete as possible. Organise how you have shown your learning steps and your standards of practice so that it is indexed and cross-referenced to the relevant sections of the paperwork. Discuss the contents of your portfolio with a colleague or a mentor to gain other people's perspectives of your work and look for blind spots.

Include evidence of your competence including any specialist expertise

You may have a particular expertise or special interest in a clinical field or non-clinical area such as management, teaching or research. It may be that you have a lead role or responsibility in your deanery, hospital or department for a specific area of care, education, research or management.

Although in hospital practice there are accreditation processes for specialist skills (*see* Chapter 4), there is little consistency in extent of training or qualifications at present within or across the various specialty areas for practitioners with a special interest (PwSI).[12] Whatever your role or responsibility or expertise, your portfolio should include examples of evidence that show that you are competent, and that you have a consistently good performance in your specialty area. You may have parallel appraisals that you can include from your employer – for example, the university if you have a research or teaching post, or a hospital consultant if he or she supervises you in the clinical specialty.

When you gather evidence of your performance at work, try to document as many aspects of your work at one time as you can, so that for example an audit covers as many of the key headings from *Good Medical Practice* (*see* Box 1.1) as possible. When you are identifying what you need to learn, or gaps in service delivery, make sure that you involve patients and show how you interact with the team. This gives you evidence about 'relationships with patients' and 'working with colleagues' as well as the clinical area you are focusing on or auditing.

Focus your cycles of evidence to your priority areas for personal development

If you are a junior doctor in training your training goals will dictate where you should focus effort. If you are a consultant, you may consider a particular local service area requires development; you may wish to develop local junior doctor professional training or initiate a research project. If you are a GP you may wish to link your cycles of evidence to service developments rewarded by the new GMS Contract or Personal Medical Services (PMS) arrangements.[13] Whatever your particular priorities you should find the following chapters will help you gain the most from your PDP, supporting you during training and preparing you for appraisal and revalidation.

References

1 Wakley G, Chambers R and Field S (2000) *Continuing Professional Development in Primary Care.* Radcliffe Medical Press, Oxford.

2 Royal College of Obstetricians and Gynaecologists (2002) *Revalidation in Obstetrics and Gynaecology Criteria, Standards and Evidence.* Royal College of Obstetricians and Gynaecologists Press, London.

3   Royal College of General Practitioners/General Practitioners Committee (2002) *Good Medical Practice for General Practitioners.* Royal College of General Practitioners, London.

4   General Medical Council (2001) *Good Medical Practice.* General Medical Council, London.

5   Department of Health (1998) *A First Class Service.* Department of Health, London.

6   Department of Health (1999) *Supporting Doctors, Protecting Patients.* Department of Health, London.

7   General Medical Council website, GMC, London. www.gmc-uk.org/revalidation

8   Mohanna K, Wall D and Chambers R (2003) *Teaching Made Easy: a manual for health professionals* (2e). Radcliffe Medical Press, Oxford.

9   Royal College of General Practitioners (1993) *Portfolio-based Learning in General Practice.* Occasional Paper 63, Royal College of General Practitioners, London.

10 Challis M (1999) AMEE Medical education guide No 11 (revised): portfolio-based learning and assessment in medical education. *Medical Teacher.* **21**: 370–86.

11 Chambers C, Wakley G, Field S and Ellis S (2003) *Appraisal for the Apprehensive.* Radcliffe Medical Press, Oxford.

12 Practitioners with a special interest website. www.gpwsi.org

13 General Practitioners Committee/The NHS Confederation (2003) *New GMS Contract. Investing in general practice.* General Practitioners Committee/NHS Confederation, London.

2

Training the trainer*

Your professional requirements as a medical teacher

The GMC[1] and the Royal Colleges have described the roles, qualities and skills of a doctor who is a competent teacher. Every doctor who is formally appointed to provide clinical or educational supervision for a doctor in training, or who undertakes to provide clinical training or supervision for medical students, should demonstrate the following personal and professional attributes:

- a commitment to the professional guidance in *Good Medical Practice* from the GMC[1]
- an enthusiasm for his/her specialty
- a personal commitment to teaching and learning
- sensitivity and responsiveness to the educational needs of students and junior doctors
- the capacity to promote development of the required professional attitudes and values
- an understanding of the principles of education as applied to medicine
- an understanding of research method
- practical teaching skills
- a willingness to develop both as a doctor and as a teacher
- a commitment to audit and peer review of his/her teaching
- the ability to use formative assessment for the benefit of the student/trainee
- the ability to carry out formal appraisal of a medical student's progress/the performance of the trainee as a practising doctor.

Focusing your trainees' learning

The Conference of Postgraduate Medical Deans (CoPMeD) proposes a model that describes the potential in every contact between trainee and trainer (*see* Box 2.1).[2]

*Much of this chapter has been adapted from Mohanna K, Wall D and Chambers R (2003) *Teaching Made Easy: a manual for health professionals* (2e). Radcliffe Medical Press, Oxford.

Box 2.1:   CoPMeD model for contact between trainee and trainer[2]
- Learning from the current patient or clinical opportunity
- Building on previous learning experience
- Opportunistic education, training and learning
- Modification of learning behaviour

Education for doctors and others working for the NHS must become more focused and relevant to the needs of the learner, patients and the NHS as a whole.[3] Multiprofessional and needs-based training is being seen as essential rather than desirable if the NHS workforce is to have 'the capacity, skills, diversity and flexibility to meet the demands on the service' that are envisaged as being integral to delivering the programme of modernisation of the NHS.[4]

As a teacher you should help individual doctors to design PDPs that address their professional requirements and also complement the overall business and development plans of their trust to deliver central and district priorities. You will help your junior doctors to optimise opportunities for learning, building on the criteria for successful learning listed in Box 2.2.[5]

Box 2.2:   Criteria for successful learning[5]
The most successful CPD involves learning which:

- is based on what is already known by the learner
- is led by the learner's own identified needs
- involves active participation by the learner
- uses the learner's own resources
- includes relevant and timely feedback
- includes self-assessment.

Insist on adult learning

Doctors are expected to be 'adult learners'. This means that to a greater or lesser extent they will be independent and self-directed. Adult learning theory is built on five assumptions:[6]

- adults are independent and self-directing
- they have accumulated a great deal of experience, which is a rich resource for learning
- they value learning that integrates with the demands of their everyday life

- they are more interested in immediate, problem-centred approaches than in subject-centred ones
- they are more motivated to learn by internal drivers than by external ones.

Medicine covers far too big a field for all the content to be delivered by us as teachers. What we need to strive for is to fit our learners up with the skills to problem solve and continue learning throughout their careers:

> Education teaches us to solve problems, the nature of which may not be known to us at the time the education is taking place and the solutions to which cannot be seen or even imagined by our teachers.[7]

Many people talk about adult learning and are frustrated by learners that: 'do not behave as adults, but expect to be spoon fed'. Underlying this frustration is often a failure to recognise that the capacity to be self-directed is not an all-or-nothing function that develops overnight. Learners act at different levels or stages of self-direction depending on many things such as previous teaching, learning and especially assessment experiences, the subject matter and the context of learning. Not all learners are ready to take responsibility for their own learning.

Effective teachers recognise this and do not just leave the learner to get on with learning entirely on their own. It is essential that adult learning is facilitated by the teacher. The trick is to match your level of delivery with the same level of self-direction the learner has reached, and try to challenge them to move to a greater degree of independence, as appropriate, depending on the subject matter.

Knowles has defined seven fundamentals that have stood the test of time as guidelines to encourage adult learners (*see* Box 2.3).[6]

Box 2.3: Fundamental guidelines for encouraging adult learners[6]

1 Establish an effective learning climate where learners feel safe and comfortable expressing themselves.
2 Involve learners in mutual planning of relevant methods and curricular content.
3 Trigger internal motivation by involving learners in diagnosing their own needs.
4 Give learners more control by encouraging them to formulate their own learning objectives.
5 Encourage learners to identify resources and devise strategies for using the resources to achieve their objectives.
6 Support learners in carrying out their learning plans.
7 Develop their skills of critical reflection by involving learners in evaluating their own learning.

Some of the most respected work on adult learners has been done by Brookfield. He lists six principles of adult learning on which we might try to build our teaching (*see* Box 2.4).[8]

Box 2.4:   Six principles of adult learning[8]

1   *Participation is voluntary*: the decision to learn is that of the learner.
2   *There should be mutual respect*: by teachers and learners of each other and by learners of other learners.
3   *Collaboration is important*: between learners and teachers and among learners.
4   *Action and reflection*: learning is a continuous process of investigation, exploration, action, reflection and further action.
5   *Critical reflection*: brings awareness that alternatives can be presented as challenges to the learner to gather evidence, ask questions and develop a critically aware frame of mind.
6   *Self-directed adult individuals need nurturing.*

We talk about developing our trainees (and ourselves!) into self-directed, independent adult learners. Knowing the principles behind the concept should help to facilitate this in real life. What can the busy consultant do to help themselves and their trainees in this respect? Brookfield gave ten tips on doing this, which are summarised in Box 2.5.[8]

Box 2.5:   How to create an adult learner[8]

1   Progressively reduce the learner's dependence on the teachers.
2   Help the learner to understand the use of learning resources including the experiences of others including fellow learners.
3   Help learners use reflective practice to define their learning needs.
4   Help learners define their learning objectives, plan their programmes and assess their own progress.
5   Organise what is to be learnt in terms of personal understanding, goals and concerns at the learners' level of understanding.
6   Encourage the learners to take decisions, to expand their learning experiences and range of opportunities for learning.
7   Encourage the use of criteria for judging all aspects of learning and not just those that are easy to measure.
8   Facilitate problem posing and problem solving in relation to personal and group needs issues.
9   Reinforce the concept of the learner as a learner with progressive mastery of skills, through constructive feedback and mutual support.
10   Emphasise experiential learning (learning by doing, learning on the job) and the use of learning contracts.

Establishing an educational climate

Educational climate may be subdivided into three parts:

1 *the physical environment*: facilities, comfort, safety, food, shelter etc
2 *the emotional climate*: security, positive methods, reinforcement etc
3 *the intellectual climate*: learning with patients, reflective practice, evidence-based, up-to-date knowledge and skills.

Remember trainees' likes and dislikes about educational climate:

- likes include:
  - encouragement and praise
  - learning on the job
  - discussing cases: including best management practice, a chance to present the case and describe their management
  - challenge
  - a relaxed atmosphere
  - group discussions
  - positive feedback
  - approachable seniors who are up to date, enthusiastic about their subject and able to say 'I do not know, let's look it up'
- dislikes include:
  - just looking at mistakes
  - humiliation especially in front of patients and staff
  - being shouted at
  - being frightened
  - teachers not appreciating that they have knowledge gaps
  - irrelevant teaching on rare conditions
  - senior colleagues who are out of date and unable to admit that they do not know everything.

Understanding the educational cycle

In hospital practice the learning agreement both for specialist registrars and the preregistration house officer assessment package is founded on this four-step model:

1 assessing the individual's needs
2 setting educational objectives
3 choosing and using a variety of methods of teaching and learning
4 assessing that learning has occurred.

Assessing the individual's needs

What does the learner need to know? Remember that you will need to assess what the trainee has done before and knows about already. You might encourage the trainee to use a tool to rate their own self-assessed levels of knowledge and skills in various areas. Using this, you may agree with your trainee some key topics they need to know and do in their time with you as a teacher. You are now ready to progress to the next step of the cycle.

Setting educational objectives·

Educational objectives are often defined as: 'things that the learner will be able to do at the end of the course, often written in behavioural terms'. For many educational activities in medicine, the objectives model fits very well, particularly in terms of practical skills. Once both trainee and educational supervisor have looked at the curriculum and have assessed needs they can devise a plan listing a set of learning objectives to achieve within the training programme. These should be written down and agreed by both parties as part of the learning agreement.

Choosing and using a variety of methods

No single method of teaching is the best. Different methods suit different situations and different learners and teachers. There are also good and not so good ways of teaching different things. It is very difficult to teach and learn communication skills on a lecture-based course. Resuscitation and suturing, for example, are best taught and learnt using simulators and mannequins to learn and practise on before having a go on real patients. Most people learn best by 'doing', using active methods of learning rather than sitting passively in a lecture theatre for a day listening to a series of keynote lectures.

Assessment

How do you know whether the trainee has learnt? One simple way is to base your assessments on the learning objectives set at the beginning of the learning process. If you have set up good achievable learning objectives and chosen appropriate learning methods, you will see the trainee progress through the course and he or she will have learnt what you expected at the beginning by the end of the course. So set learning objectives at the start, check progress as you go along by regular appraisal meetings and assess completion of learning at the end.

Giving feedback effectively

Constructive feedback is the art of holding conversations with learners about their performance. It has two elements: it should contain enough specific detail and advice to enable the recipient to reflect and enhance their practice and it should be positive and supportive in tone. There is some evidence that constructive feedback can improve learning outcomes and enable students to develop a deep approach to their learning with the active pursuit of understanding and application of knowledge, rather than adopting a superficial approach. It can improve competence at least in the short term.[9]

It is important that as well as being positive in tone (for reasons of self-esteem, morale and the development of good communication skills by observation of the teacher), there should be a balance between comment on areas to improve and feedback that is positive in content. You should aim to give feedback about deficiencies and strengths. The skill of the effective teacher is to find the balance between support and challenge, and the best feedback is high on support and high on challenge. Box 2.6 describes the qualities of feedback of different dimensions. The best way to learn how to give effective feedback is to practise it.

Box 2.6: Qualities of feedback

High support

'That was great, you're obviously trying hard.' *Safe, general, potentially patronising*	'A good effort. I could see how you were drawing the feelings out – I wonder if you got to the crux of the matter?' *Focused, attentive, potentially threatening*

Low challenge   **High challenge**

'Good. Carry on. Seems to be working.' *In passing, nothing specific, dismissive*	'Well that could have been better – why did you not focus more early on?' *Critical, induces defensiveness, potentially paralysing*

Low support

There is one golden rule: give positive praise of things that have been well done first. General rules:

- focus on behaviour rather than interpretation
- give specific examples
- aim to be descriptive or sensory based rather then interpretive, non-sensory based
- aim to be non-judgemental rather then evaluative.

Examples are shown in Table 2.1.

Table 2.1:   Giving feedback

Evaluative, interpretive or judgemental	Descriptive, sensory based
'The beginning was awful, you just seemed to ignore her.'	'At the start you were looking at the notes, which prevented eye contact.'
'The beginning was excellent, great stuff.'	'At the beginning you gave her your full attention and never lost eye contact – your facial expression registered interest in what she was saying.'
'It's no good getting embarrassed when patients talk about their sexual history.'	'I noticed you were very flushed when she spoke about her husband's impotence, and you lost eye contact ...'

Assessment

The word assessment is used for the processes and instruments applied to measure the learner's achievements, normally after they have worked through a learning programme of one sort or another.

Assessment is a hurdle to be passed to allow progress to the next stage. This is 'pass' or 'fail', and is usually called 'summative' assessment by educationalists i.e. it 'sums up' achievement at the end of a period of study. (This distinguishes it from formative assessment that 'informs' you of achievements as you go along, highlighting progress and areas to develop while there is still time to do something about it, otherwise known as appraisal – *see* Chapter 1. Senior house officers and specialist registrars have appraisal with educational supervisors.)

The link between aims and objectives and assessment

The first step in designing an assessment tool is in curriculum development as you set your aims and objectives.

- *Aims* are broad statements of intent. For example, you might aim to produce a competent doctor in reproductive health. They specify the broad direction in which you want your learner to go; they do not specify how far they have to go or how they will get there or how they will know when they are there.
- *Objectives* are outcomes measures, and are much more specific statements addressed at aspects of the aim. They are usually written in terms of what the learner will be able to do at the end of the course of study.

It is surprising how often people set out to teach without having a clear idea in mind of exactly what they are planning to achieve. They decide, for example, to have a tutorial on 'egg sharing'. From the teacher's perspective, without clear objectives it is impossible to choose the teaching method best able to deliver the subject matter, to know what content can be left out and what is vital, to be sure whether the course has worked or how to evaluate it. From the learner's perspective, clear objectives, framed as learning outcomes, help them decide whether a course of study is for them and will suit their learning needs, help plan their study, choose what aspects to go into in depth and how to prepare for assessments.

Domains of learning[10]

These may simply be thought of as:

* knowledge
* skills
* attitudes.

To be clear about what we are asking our learners to learn about, we need to consider which domain we are assessing and at which level. A taxonomy is a hierarchical and orderly classification in which each stage builds on the one above. For example, each domain, proceeding from the simple to the complex, can be subdivided as in Table 2.2. The effective domain proceeds from aspects outside the learner to more internal processes.

Table 2.2: Subdivision of domains of learning

Level	Domain		
	Knowledge	*Skills*	*Attitudes*
Base level	1 Knowledge 2 Comprehension	1 Observation 2 Imitation	1 Receiving (Listening) 2 Responding
Application	3 Application	3 Practising	3 Valuing (Advocating Defending)
Problem solving	4 Analysis 5 Synthesis 6 Evaluation	4 Mastering 5 Adapting	4 Organisation 5 Characterisation (Judging)

Assessments: desirable criteria[11]

You should strive for certain principles in assessment to help you to be as fair as possible. The as near to 'ideal' as possible assessment should be:

* *valid*: it measures what it is supposed to measure (if it has face validity as well, it also looks to the learner as though it is measuring what it purports to measure)
* *reliable*: it measures it with essentially the same result each time (learners with the same level of performance will be judged equally regardless of who administers it)
* *practicable*: it is easy to do in terms of cost, time and skills of the assessors
* *fair to the learners and the teachers*: e.g. differences between learners that are irrelevant to the subject being assessed do not affect the result, marking is not unnecessarily burdensome for teachers
* *useful to the learners and the teachers*: e.g. it discriminates between good and poor candidates
* *acceptable*: in terms of, for example, cultural and gender issues
* *appropriate*: to what has been taught and learnt on the programme.

Sometimes there is a trade off between validity and reliability; increase in one is often at the expense of the other. Consider multiple choice question (MCQ) assessments for communication skills; they are very reliable, equally performing learners will score equally, but are likely to have low validity. The extent to which they can measure communication skills is low. At the other extreme we can increase validity by introducing simulated (or real) patients but reliability will fall off; we cannot be sure that learners of similar ability will score the same across all the simulated patients.

Being a good supervisor

An educational supervisor works with the learner to develop and facilitate an educational plan that addresses their educational needs. Ideally educational supervision should be focused on educational development and be separate from supervision of clinical practice or remedial help for underperformance. This is rarely possible in practice and an educational supervisor usually has multiple responsibilities for a trainee. They may be expected to give support, facilitate education and training, supervise educational progress, supervise clinical work, provide and co-ordinate service-based training, provide support for formal educational programmes, provide pastoral and careers counselling and may represent the employer.

The educational supervisor should agree a structured personal educational plan with the learner dependent on the learner's needs and aspirations. The supervisor will usually maintain an overview of the learner's performance and career progress.

The role of the educational supervisor is to provide:[12]

- professional and personal support for the trainee
- facilitation of education and training
- supervision of the trainee's educational progress
- supervision of the trainee's clinical work as appropriate
- co-ordinated service-based training
- support for a formal educational programme
- signposting to pastoral and careers counselling as required
- good employer practice – ensuring a clear job description/training prospectus for each post (if the learner is an employee).

The checklist in Box 2.7 describes how good educational supervisors will interact with their trainees.

Box 2.7: A good educational supervisor should:
- meet with the learner early in the post and help with the induction to the post
- agree aims and objectives for learning in the post
- construct the learning agreement with the learner
- give feedback on progress to the learner
- discuss career aims and the training programme
- assess the learner at the end of the post on their learning objectives
- give feedback to the teacher on the training posts and programmes (if appropriate).

The challenging trainee

Sometimes it all goes wrong. You have tried everything and are still up against it with a trainee who is not learning or performing well. Sometimes the difficulty lies with the trainee, sometimes with you as the teacher and sometimes the trainee–teacher relationship. There are probably as many causes of this as there are challenging trainees, but there are some recurring themes. Issues may include mismatch between style of teaching and the stage of self-directedness of the trainee, mismatch of learning style between the trainee and the teacher, problems with learning-group dynamics, health-related issues (both physical and mental), stress, problems outside of work such as family difficulties or illness, and disciplinary matters.

Difficulties show themselves in many ways:

- non-attendance for teaching sessions
- non-participation in groups or destructive group behaviour
- not keeping up to date or preparing for teaching
- failure in exams
- tardiness or failure to turn up for work
- incomplete tasks during work time, not answering their bleep
- problems with working in the team
- inability to take or give instructions to staff
- poor communication with, or complaints from, patients.

These are all symptoms of underlying difficulties and it can help to ask:

- what is the real problem?
- why has this happened now?
- what can we do about it?
- can we get back on course?

Just as in clinical practice the treatment is less likely to work if the diagnosis is wrong, measures aimed at symptoms may not address the real difficulty. There are certain general principles that may help when addressing concerns about trainees:

- *do it now*: tackle the problem when it occurs and not at the end of the placement
- *explain the problem*: explore the issues with learner, ask for their views or comments and plan how to get back on course
- *give support*: and encouragement
- *document what you do*: appraisals, assessments, comments from others, incidents etc and keep copies of all paperwork. Use the correct framework as laid down by your specialty training committee or Royal College or professional organisation
- *share the problem*: do not try to do it all on your own but get advice from others – other teachers, educational supervisors, your specialty tutor, your clinical tutor, your own line manager, the training programme director, chair of your specialty training committee or the postgraduate dean's office
- *inform*: senior colleagues as appropriate.

Having explored the issue, ask yourself:

- is this an educational issue that the trainee and I can tackle between us and with the tools available to us?
- is this a relationship problem or personality clash between the trainee and me?
- do I need help from someone else to help guide this trainee?

- does the trainee need careers advice? Are they in the wrong career?
- does the trainee (or me as teacher) have other problems such as stress, physical or mental illness etc?

If it is not possible to get back on track

You may conclude alone, or in discussion with the trainee, that the situation is beyond your joint capacity to solve. It might be that just transferring to another educational supervisor, intermitting from the course to return later or changing career direction is what is needed. Good teachers respond positively to these situations, as it should not be taken as a sign of failure but rather one of maturity, to recognise the limitations of a situation and know how to go about addressing them.

The following areas might help you decide where to turn next for help.

Does the trainee need to be referred to occupational health or a doctor?

It is important in all teaching relationships to recognise the explicit and implicit boundaries. This is especially important in the healthcare professions when it is easy to slip into the role of problem solver or caregiver.

Try to recognise when you are acting as a health adviser. If this happens, ensure your trainees have a GP to consult and know how to signpost them to occupational health if need be. This makes sure they get impartial advice and protects you from a charge that you colluded in an issue that may have put patients at risk. If a trainee is better off not at work, you might not give the same advice as their own doctor who is not also their line manager, or if they plead with you to continue at work because the exams are coming up.

Issues that might come up are acute illnesses, flare-ups of chronic conditions, drug or alcohol dependence, counselling for depression or anxiety. Issuing prescriptions or offering quick sessions of acupuncture or chiropractic between teaching sessions are best avoided!

Does the trainee need to see a careers counsellor?

What if the trainee thinks that he or she is a square peg in a round hole? Or what if you have come to that conclusion and they cannot see it yet? What if the onset of a degenerative disease is limiting their career options? The advisory skills required in this area are specialised. Most people working in medicine have invested a lot in terms of time and commitment to getting where they are now, it may be the result of a lifelong career plan, and the thought of changing direction can be daunting.

You need to raise this with the trainee and seek their opinions. If they agree, consider putting them in touch with specialist career counsellors.

Is this a disciplinary matter?

Sometimes these can be the easiest issues to deal with if trainees are guilty of obvious breaches of the implicit code of conduct such as fraud, theft or violent behaviour. In clear and significant breaches, such as persistently being under the influence of alcohol at work, all professional groups have made it an obligation on members to protect the public from incompetent or dangerous practitioners, and part of being a professional is to be aware of that obligation to report such practitioners to our regulatory bodies.

Deciding whether to institute disciplinary proceedings is a difficult decision to take and one that most teachers should not be taking on their own. Always discuss such problems with colleagues either formally or informally to gain a second opinion or advice.

As an illustration of the routes available, consider the example in Box 2.8 below.

Box 2.8: The West Midlands regional postgraduate dean's policy for handling disciplinary matters in hospital practice

Disciplinary matters sometimes overlap with educational problems, so you do need to be clear about what is going on. The West Midlands policy divides the areas into three as described below.

1 *Personal conduct*: the trust must take the lead, take action under local guidelines and inform the Department of Postgraduate Medical and Dental Education (PMDE). An example of such a matter in this category would be theft of hospital property or assault on another member of staff.
2 *Professional conduct*: the trust should take the lead, involve the PMDE from the start, and decide jointly with them on what action is to be taken. An example of such a matter in this category would be a breach of patient confidentiality.
3 *Professional competence*: this is the principal responsibility of the PMDE, but they should keep the trust informed of the actions to be taken. An example of such a matter in this category might be a doctor or dentist performing a clinical task badly, with a poor outcome. Inevitably there will be training and supervision issues also.

Grievance procedures

Sometimes the trainee doctor will be aggrieved by some action you take or feel that they are being harassed. They may feel you have unfairly assessed their work or given them an inaccurate reference. They may invoke the grievance procedure laid down in the trust's contract of employment. If you are unfortunate enough to be involved in such a process, seek help and advice as soon as you become aware of the issue.

* If the trainee makes a formal grievance action, the employing trust's procedures must be followed.
* For informal grievance procedures against educational supervisors or mentors, the regional dean should be involved if the trainee is a doctor or dentist or your professional body should be contacted for other professional groups.

References

1 General Medical Council (2001) *Good Medical Practice.* General Medical Council, London.

2 The Conference of Postgraduate Medical Deans (CoPMeD) ad hoc working group on the educational implications of the European working time directive (2002*) Liberating Learning: a practical guide for learners and teachers to postgraduate medical education and the European working time directive.* CoPMeD, London.

3 Houghton G and Wall D (1999) Clinical governance and the Chief Medical Officer's review of GP education: piecing the New NHS jigsaw together. *Medical Teacher.* **21(1):** 5–6.

4 National Health Service Executive (1998) *Working Together. Securing a quality workforce for the NHS.* Department of Health, London.

5 Roland M, Holden J and Campbell S (1999) *Quality Assessment for General Practice: supporting clinical governance in primary care groups.* National Primary Care Research and Development Centre, University of Manchester.

6 Knowles MS (1984) *Androgogy in Action: applying modern principles of adult learning.* Jossey-Bass, San Francisco.

7 Marinker M (1992) Assessment of postgraduate medical education – future directions. In: M Lawrence and P Pritchard (eds) *General Practice Education UK and Nordic Perspectives.* Springer Verlag, London.

8 Brookfield SD (1986) *Understanding and Facilitating Adult Learning.* Open University Press, Milton Keynes.

9   Rolfe I and McPherson J (1995) Formative assessment: how am I doing? *Lancet.* **345:** 37–9.

10 Bloom BS (1956) *Taxonomy of Educational Objectives 1. Cognitive domain.* David McKay, New York.

11 Wakeford R (1999) Principles of assessment. In: H Fry, S Ketteridge and S Marshall (eds) (1999) *Teaching and Learning in Higher Education.* Kogan Page, London.

12 Department of Postgraduate Medical and Dental Education South and West (1997) *Education Supervision: a handbook for hospital based educational support.* PGMDE, South and West Region.

Further reading

• Mohanna K, Wall D and Chambers R (2003) *Teaching Made Easy: a manual for health professionals* (2e). Radcliffe Medical Press, Oxford.

3

Methods of effective learning

Most people learn best through experiential learning: learning through doing rather than passively receiving.[1] Effective learning also involves learning through reflecting on what you have done.[2] The learner's previous experience plays an important role in that you are building on and adding to established knowledge and skills. So read through this section and reflect on it from your own perspective, and also from that of the juniors and colleagues you teach, to help them learn more effectively too.

Ways of learning

Using variety in acquiring new information or skills helps you to utilise your time with maximum efficiency. Identify your dominant learning style (*see* Table 3.1) but recognise that, if you use as many different learning methods as you can, they reinforce each other.[3] To maximise the learning when you are working alone:

- tick off each section as you read it, or when you understand it
- highlight or emphasise new information
- read the important points dramatically, or whisper them
- summarise the material out loud
- visualise the material internally
- walk around while reading or listening
- put key ideas on post-it notes and arrange them in different meaningful patterns on your desk, board, or wall
- make notes of your own thoughts, generating your own version
- go for a walk and reflect on what you have been reading.

Table 3.1: Learning styles

Read the situations in the left column and then choose which column contains the most options that suit you. This will be your dominant style of learning.

Situation	Visual	Auditory	Action
When you cannot spell a word, do you:	try and visualise the word?	sound out the word?	write down the word to see if feels right?
Talking: do you use words like:	see, picture, imagine?	hear, tune, think?	feel, touch, hold?
Are you distracted by:	looking at your surroundings or by untidiness?	sounds and noises?	activity and movement?
You prefer to contact people:	face to face or by writing?	by telephone?	while walking or participating in an activity?
You remember people best when you recall:	where you met or what they were wearing?	what you talked about?	what you were doing?
When reading do you prefer:	descriptive scenes or to imagine the scene?	dialogue or plays?	lots of action, to do things rather than reading?
When you do something new at work do you prefer to have:	a demonstration or see it written on a poster or diagram?	verbal instructions or talk it through with someone?	to try it out yourself?
When you are assembling something do you prefer to:	look at the directions and pictures?	have someone to read out the directions?	just put it together and only use the directions if you are stuck?
If you need help with a computer programme you:	look for pictures or diagrams?	phone a help line or ask someone?	keep trying different ways?

Explore from different angles

There are additional ways in which you might be able to bring your particular type of learning styles into play. Try looking at the material in different ways that are related to them:

• describe the material out loud, or use question and answer format
• use a flowchart or diagram for the material
• make an image or a model of the material

- play background music as you learn, or sing important points aloud
- teach someone else
- reflect on the material
- use index cards with important points sorted in different ways.

Make the task manageable

You may also find it helpful to organise things into parcels of particular sizes. If you feel overwhelmed by a particular task, try breaking it down into smaller sections. On another occasion, you may feel irritated by the detail involved in trying to achieve something, so that you need to be able to draw back and see how it fits into a bigger picture.

It's also a good idea to put the things you see into a framework to connect them to what you already know. It doesn't much matter in which direction you build this framework, but the existence of the structure increases your feeling that you are in control of this new material, makes it feel less overwhelming and reduces the amount of explicit content you have to remember.

Show you know

Demonstrating to yourself that you really do understand and remember can increase your confidence that your learning is really working. Teaching someone else, writing about new information or demonstrating new skills can reinforce your learning and confidence.

Review and reflect on the process

After a learning session, review the process you followed. Look at what worked, what didn't, and what you would do differently next time. At the end of a lecture or workshop session, use the feedback sheets to reflect on what went well, what didn't and why that was. Make notes of what you've learned about learning, and use them to improve your next learning activity.

Develop a strong work ethic

There is no such thing as a lazy excellent doctor. You do not have to be brilliant to be competent but you do have to have the persistence and determination to keep working at it.

Don't procrastinate

You need to set aside time to achieve competency. Time is spent reading, reflecting on reviewing notes, talking to colleagues, working on tasks on your own or with others, obtaining advice from the tutors, and going to educational and training sessions. Develop the habit of always making a note when you come across something you don't know, so that if you cannot look it up, or ask about it at the time, you can do so later. Time management is one of the most difficult tasks of learning. Life is full with doing clinical work, or administration, having a home life or social time. Learning and reflecting on what you are doing tend to be squeezed out.

Set your priorities

If you are required to know about specific areas or to be competent in particular skills, these will be high up on your priority list. It is very tempting just to learn about the things that interest you or that you find easy. Establish your learning needs, not desires (*see* also page 38).

Get used to working in groups and teams

Have a group of people with whom you can study. Everyone approaches complex problems differently, so working with a team may allow someone to see an aspect of the problem that they would otherwise not consider. Everything that you change needs the co-operation of others in your team, so make sure that you involve them in appreciating that a problem exists and with working out and applying the possible solutions. You are likely to have blind spots and working with others and getting their feedback will help identify your gaps.

Don't rely on group work to do everything for you

The problems never look that difficult when you see the solutions developed by your group or team members or tutors and facilitators. The solutions appear straightforward and relatively short. However, the amount of trial and error and flipping through notes and books that it takes to develop those answers is actually immense and often shared between many people. When you are on your own, you need to be able to come up with answers on your own from all the information you have learnt so far. This can be difficult or impossible if you have relied on your group to do your thinking for you.

Be organised

This applies to everything from taking notes to solving problems. You should be able to find the information that you spent so long retrieving and be able to read and understand it. You should be able to look at a problem you worked on and know what you were doing and why. Invest in reference manager software so that you can easily track down that elusive reference. Keep your files – paper or computer – labelled clearly and keep back-ups.

Use the resources available

Make sure that you know who can help you find things out – the librarian, the secretary, colleagues or the tutor. Use the internet and the library. Read journals and arrange for email alerts for the subjects you need to keep up to date.

Recognise that you have to train your brain to think differently

Many people think the way to do well is to understand a little bit more or memorise more information. In lifelong learning, what is important is not memorising stuff but the way you think and apply what you have learnt in your everyday working life. Retrain the brain to think about how to apply concepts. You might find the concept of competence easier to understand as levels of competence.

The levels of knowledge and skills can be graded as follows:[4]

1 *not relevant to post*
2 *novice*: knows a little about the topic and has not generally given advice about the topic or performed work associated with it
3 *advanced beginner*: has some knowledge about the subject; is able to direct people to appropriate services; is able to give a limited amount of advice about the subject
4 *competent*: has a good basic knowledge about the topic and how to apply it at work, and is able to demonstrate this knowledge and skills to others
5 *proficient*: has a wide knowledge and is skilled in the subject; deals with situations presented on a daily basis, advising, treating and managing people and referring to others when applicable

6   *expert*: has an 'enormous background of experience', and 'intuitive grasp of each situation'; interprets and synthesises information and can handle a wide range of problems in different contexts.

Set yourself achievable targets

Talk through what you have set yourself to do with at least one other person and check that you have made it sufficiently simple and achievable. Build in staging posts to measure how well you are doing on the way to your goal. If you find you are trying to do too much in too short a time, revise your objectives and postpone some of the task to later.

Maintain the right state of mind

If you think about a situation where you seemed to soak up knowledge without any real effort, you will probably find that all of the aspects listed below came into play, so apply them when you have something that you have to do.

1   Find a personal reason why you want to want to learn this material or skill. This may be something that's already clear in your mind, but it may be something that you have to create. Creating a desire to learn something specific may require connecting the knowledge to your self-image; it may help to think in terms of missing skills that you would like to have; or you may need to connect the knowledge to your larger goals. However, if you don't have a good reason to learn, learning will not happen easily and may not happen at all. You can't be compelled to learn.

2   Having come up with your reasons for learning something, you need to translate these reasons into motivation. Asking questions like 'what's in it for me?' may help. For most people, increasing the emotional content of the reason adds extra motivation. Try to visualise, hear, or feel some situation that will result from having learnt the material.

3   Find a way to make the material relevant to you, right now. One way to do this is to ask, 'what's most important about this material?' or 'how can I use this material now?' Connect the material or skill to things that you know already. Then practise using the knowledge or skill. Learning something and then putting it into use is one of the most effective ways of learning (experiential learning).

4   Build up anticipation about learning the material. Imagine what insights might come to you when you really understand the material. Imagine passing an examination easily. Imagine being able to answer a technical question well at a job interview. Imagine feeling confident that you can

demonstrate your competence at your appraisal. Whatever it takes, find a way to want to get started.

5   Have positive expectations: that you will find the material easy to understand, that it will be interesting, that it will be exciting, that it will be useful, that it will connect with what you already know. Expectations are self-fulfilling prophecies – what you expect is what you get.

Learning is fun and can give you a real buzz of excitement as you realise that you achieve new knowledge or apply a new skill.

Setting standards to show that you are competent

Doctors 'must be committed to lifelong learning and be responsible for maintaining the medical knowledge and clinical and team skills necessary for the provision of quality care'.[5]

You could make a good start by describing your roles and responsibilities. This will help you to define what your competence should be now, or what competence you are hoping to attain (for instance as a GP with a special interest (GPwSI)). Once you have your definition, you can recognise whether you have, or lack in some part, the necessary competence. If there are no accepted descriptions of competence in the area you are focusing on, then you will have to start from scratch. You might compile your description from national guidelines such as in the National Service Frameworks or health strategies. Usually you can find guidance about competency from specialist sources such as associations for clinical topics or the various Royal Colleges. The Department of Health in England has worked with the Royal College of General Practitioners (RCGP) to describe the competency of GPwSIs in many clinical areas.[6]

A good definition of competence is someone who is: 'able to perform the tasks and roles required to the expected standard'.[7]

You will need to describe the standards expected in the range of tasks and roles you undertake and reference the source of standard setting. If professionals, or their organisations, are the only people involved in setting those standards, consider whether you should amend or extend the standards, tasks or roles by considering other perspectives such as those of patients or the NHS as a whole.

There is a difference between being competent, and performing in a consistently competent manner. You need to be motivated to perform consistently well and enabled to do so with efficient systems and sufficient resources. You will require sufficient numbers of other competent doctors or staff and available infrastructure such as diagnostic and treatment resources.[8]

Choose methods in Stage 3 (*see* Chapter 1) to demonstrate your standards of performance and identify any learning needs that span different topic areas, to reduce duplication and maximise the usefulness of your learning. Collecting evidence of more than one aspect of your competence or performance cuts down the overall amount of work underpinning your PDP or included in your appraisal portfolio.

Use several methods to identify your learning needs and/or gaps in your service development or delivery, so that you validate the findings of one method by another. No one method will give you reliable information about the gaps in your knowledge, skills or attitudes or everyday service. Does what you think about your performance match with what others in the team or patients think of how you practise in your everyday work? It is particularly difficult to determine what it is you 'don't know you don't know' by yourself, yet it is vital that you identify and rectify those gaps. Other people may be able to tell you what you need to learn quite readily. Colleagues from different disciplines could usefully comment on any shortfalls in how your work interfaces with theirs.

Patients or people who don't use your services could tell you whether the way you operate or provide services is off-putting or inappropriate. There may be data about your performance or that of your practice that could point out those gaps in your knowledge or skills of which you were previously unaware.

Determine what it is that you 'don't know you don't know' by:

- asking patients, users and non-users of your service
- comparing your performance against best practice or that of peers
- comparing your performance against objectives in business plans or national directives
- asking colleagues from different disciplines about shortfalls in how your work interfaces with theirs.

Stage 3A: Identify your learning needs – how you can find out if you need to be better at doing your job

You may decide to use a few selected methods to gather baseline evidence of your performance, focused on your specific area of expertise. You may target other topics or areas at the same time that are relevant to the various sections of the GMC's booklet *Good Medical Practice*.[9] For this type of combined assessment, you might use several of the methods described in this chapter such as:

- constructive feedback from peers or patients
- 360° feedback

- self-assessment, or review by others, using a rating scale to assess your skills and attitudes
- comparison with protocols and guidelines for checking how well procedures are followed
- audit: various types and applications
- significant event audit
- eliciting patient views such as satisfaction surveys
- a SWOT (strengths, weaknesses, opportunities and threats) or SCOT (strengths, challenges, opportunities and threats) analysis
- reading and reflecting
- educational review.

Seek feedback

Find colleagues who will give you constructive feedback about your performance and practice. The golden rule for giving constructive feedback is to give positive praise of things that have been well done first. Sometimes colleagues launch straight in to criticise faults when asked for their views. The Pendleton model of the giving of feedback is widely used in the health setting (*see* Box 3.1):[10]

Box 3.1:   The Pendleton model of giving feedback

1   The 'learner' goes first and performs the activity.
2   Questions from the 'teacher' clarify any facts.
3   The 'learner' says what they thought was done well.
4   The 'teacher' says what they thought was done well.
5   The 'learner' says what could be improved upon.
6   The 'teacher' says what could be improved upon.
7   Both discuss ideas for improvements in a helpful and constructive manner.

360° feedback

This collects together perceptions from a number of different participants as shown in Figure 3.1.

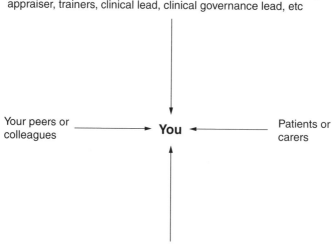

People to whom you are responsible: hospital or practice managers, appraiser, trainers, clinical lead, clinical governance lead, etc

Your peers or colleagues ——→ **You** ←—— Patients or carers

People responsible to you: clinical and non-clinical staff

Figure 3.1:   360° feedback.

The wider the spread of people giving feedback, the more rounded the picture. Each individual gives a feedback questionnaire to at least three people in each of the groups above. An independent person then collects and collates the questionnaires and discusses the results with the individual. Computerised versions are available from commercial companies.[11] The main disadvantage of this method is that it can sometimes be spoilt by malicious comments against which individuals cannot readily defend themselves.

Self-assess or gain another person's perspective on your standard of practice or service delivery

You might describe any aspect of your practice as statements (A to G as in Box 3.2) about your competence or performance for you to self-assess or others to give you feedback or comments by marking the extent to which they agree on the linear scales opposite. You could use the descriptions of an excellent GP in *Good Medical Practice for General Practitioners*[7] as we have done in relating statements in Box 3.2 to consultation skills. For instance, if statement A is: 'I consistently treat patients politely and with consideration',[12] you could self-assess the extent to which you agree. Alternatively, you could ask colleagues or patients to fill in the assessment form. Objective feedback from external assessment is usually more reliable than your own self-assessment when you may have blind spots about your own performance. As you become more confident in this method of reviewing your competence, you might emphasise how consistent you are in your application of good practice – so in the statements below we have sometimes included 'consistently', 'always' or 'usually'. You can set your own challenges. If you have a mentor or a 'buddy' at work with whom you learn, you might discuss and reflect on the completed marking grids with him or her.

Box 3.2: Marking grid: circle the number which represents your views or feelings about each statement – complete the grid on more than one occasion and compare results over time

A   I consistently treat patients politely and with consideration.

STRONGLY AGREE   to   STRONGLY DISAGREE

1----------------2----------------3----------------4----------------5---------------6

B   I am aware of how my personal beliefs could affect the care offered to the patient, and take care not to impose my own beliefs and values.

STRONGLY AGREE   to   STRONGLY DISAGREE

1----------------2----------------3----------------4----------------5---------------6

C   I always treat all patients equally and ensure that some groups are not favoured at the expense of others.

STRONGLY AGREE   to   STRONGLY DISAGREE

1----------------2----------------3----------------4----------------5---------------6

D   I try to maintain a relationship with the patient or family when a mistake has occurred.

STRONGLY AGREE   to   STRONGLY DISAGREE

1----------------2----------------3----------------4----------------5---------------6

E   I always obtain informed consent to treatment.

STRONGLY AGREE   to   STRONGLY DISAGREE

1----------------2----------------3----------------4----------------5---------------6

F   I usually involve patients in decisions about their care.

STRONGLY AGREE   to   STRONGLY DISAGREE

1----------------2----------------3----------------4----------------5---------------6

G   I always respect the right of patients to refuse treatments or tests.

STRONGLY AGREE   to   STRONGLY DISAGREE

1----------------2----------------3----------------4----------------5---------------6

Compare your performance against protocols or guidelines

Are you familiar with all the protocols or guidelines that are used by someone, somewhere at work? You might determine your learning needs and those of other team members by piling all the protocols or guidelines in a big heap and rationalising them so that you have a common set in your unit or practice. Working as a team you can compare your own knowledge and usual practice with others and with protocols or guidelines recommended by the National Institute for Clinical Excellence (NICE),[13] the National Service Frameworks, the Scottish Intercollegiate Guidelines Network (SIGN)[14] or the Royal College of Obstetricians and Gynaecologists' guidelines.[15] You could audit the standard of your practice to find out how often you adhere to such a protocol or guideline, and if you can justify why you deviate from the recommendations.

Audit

Audit is:

> the method used by health professionals to assess, evaluate, and improve the care of patients in a systematic way, to enhance their health and quality of life.[16]

The five steps of the audit cycle are shown in Box 3.3.

Box 3.3:   The five steps of the audit cycle

1   Describe the criteria and standards you are trying to achieve.
2   Measure your current performance of how well you are providing care or services in an objective way.
3   Compare your performance against criteria and standards.
4   Identify the need for change – to performance, adjustment of criteria or standards, resources, available data.
5   Make any required changes as necessary and re-audit later.

Performance or practice is often broken down for the purposes of audit into the three aspects of structure, process and outcome. Structural audits might concern resources such as equipment, premises, skills, people, etc. Process audits focus on what is done to the patient: for instance, clinical protocols and guidelines. Audits of outcomes consider the impact of care or services on the patient and might include patient satisfaction, health gains and effectiveness of care or services. You might look at aspects of quality of the structure, process and outcome of the delivery of any clinical field – focusing on access, equity of care between different groups in the population, efficiency, economy, effectiveness for individual patients, etc.[16]

Set standards for your performance, find out how you are doing, search to find out best practice, make the changes and then re-audit the care given to patients in the future with the same problem. Some variations on audit include:

- *Case note analysis.* This gives an insight into your current practice. It might be a retrospective review of a random selection of notes, or a prospective survey of consecutive patients with the same condition as they present to see you.
- *Peer review.* Compare an area of practice with other individual professionals or managers; or compare practice teams as a whole. An independent body might compare all practices in one area e.g. within a trust or organisation so that like is compared with like. Feedback may be arranged to protect participants' identities so that only the individual person or practice knows their own identity, the rest being anonymised, for example by giving each practice a number. Where there is mutual trust and an open learning culture, peer review does not need to be anonymised and everyone can learn together about making improvements in practice.
- *Criteria-based audit.* This compares clinical practice with specific standards, guidelines or protocols. Re-audit of changes should demonstrate improvements in the quality of patient care.
- *External audit.* Prescribing advisers or managers in PCOs can supply information about indicators of performance for audit. Visits from external bodies such as the Healthcare Commission expose the PCO or hospital trust in England and Wales to external audit.
- *Tracer criteria.* Assessing the quality of care of a 'tracer' condition may be used to represent the quality of care of other similar conditions or more complex problems. Tracer criteria should be easily defined and measured.

Significant event audit

Think of an incident where a patient or you experienced an adverse event. This might be an unexpected death, an unplanned pregnancy, an avoidable side-effect from prescribed medication, a violent attack on a member of staff, or an angry outburst in public by you or a work colleague. You can review the case and reflect on the sequence of events that led to that critical event occurring. It is likely that there were a multitude of factors leading up to that significant event. You should take the case to a multidisciplinary meeting to reflect and analyse what were the triggers, causes and consequences of the event. Complete the significant event audit cycle by planning what individuals or the department as a whole might do to avoid a similar event happening in future. This might include undertaking further learning and/or making appropriate changes to your systems.

The steps of a significant event audit are shown in Box 3.4.

Box 3.4:   Steps of a significant event audit

- *Step 1*: Describe who was involved, what time of day, what the task/activity was, the context and any other relevant information.
- *Step 2*: Reflect on the effects of the event on the participants and the professionals involved.
- *Step 3*: Discuss the reasons for the event or situation arising with other colleagues, review case notes or other records.
- *Step 4*: Decide how you or others might have behaved differently. Describe your options for how the procedures at work might be changed to minimise or eliminate the chances of the event recurring.
- *Step 5*: Plan changes that are needed, how they will be implemented, who will be responsible for what and when, what further training or resources are required. Then carry out the changes.
- *Step 6*: Re-audit later to see whether changes to procedures or new knowledge and skills are having the desired effects. Give feedback to the practice team.

An assessment by an external body

This is a traditional way of showing that you are competent by taking and passing an examination. It is a good way of testing recalled knowledge in a written or oral examination, or establishing how you behave in a clinical situation on the day of a practical examination, but not much good for measuring anything else. A summative examination (i.e. done at the end of a course of study) gives a measure of your learning up to that date.

You might undertake an objective test of your knowledge and skills. Examples are a computer-based test in the form of multiple choice questions and patient management problems.

Elicit the views of patients

Part of meeting the criteria for relationships with patients in *Good Medical Practice*[9] might be to assess patients' satisfaction with:

- you
- your practice
- the local hospital's way of working
- other services available in your locality.

Avoid surveys where questions are relatively superficial or biased. A more specific enquiry should uncover particular elements of patients' dissatis-faction, which will be more useful if you are trying to identify your learning needs. Use a well-validated patient questionnaire, instead of risking producing your own version with ambiguities and flaws, such as the Doctors' Inter-personal Skills Questionnaire (DISQ).[17] Many doctors and practice teams have used these patient survey methods, providing a bank of data against which to compare your performance.

Other sources of feedback from patients might be obtained through sugges-tion boxes for patients to contribute comments, or the departmental team recording all patients' suggestions and complaints however trivial, looking for patterns in the comments received.

There will be learning to be had from every complaint – even if the complaint does not have any substance, there should be something to learn about the shortfall in communication between you and the complainant.

The evolution of the 'expert patient programme' should mean that there is a pool of well informed patients with chronic conditions who can contribute their insights into what you (or the service) need to learn from a patient's perspective.[18]

Strengths, weaknesses (or challenges), opportunities and threats (SWOT or SCOT) analysis

You can undertake a SWOT (or SCOT) analysis of your own performance or that of your team or trust, working it out on your own, or with a workmate or mentor, or with a group of colleagues. Brainstorm the strengths, weaknesses (or challenges), opportunities and threats of your role or circumstances.

Strengths and weaknesses (or challenges) of your roles might relate to your clinical knowledge or skills, experience, expertise, decision making, communi-cation skills, interprofessional relationships, political skills, timekeeping, organ-isational skills, teaching skills, or research skills. Strengths and weaknesses (or challenges) of the organisation might relate to most of these aspects as well as the way resources are allocated, overall efficiency and the degree to which the organisation is patient centred.

Opportunities might relate to your unexploited experience or potential strengths, expected changes in the NHS, or resources for which you might bid. For example, you might train for and set up a special interest post.

Threats will include factors and circumstances that prevent you from achieving your aims for personal, professional and task development or service improvements. They might be to do with your health, turnover in the departmental team, or time-limited investment by the trust.

List the important factors in your SWOT (or SCOT) analysis in order of priority through discussion with colleagues and independent people from outside your workplace. Draw up goals and a timed action plan for you or the team to follow.

Informal conversations – in the corridor, over coffee

You learn such a lot when chatting with colleagues at coffee time or over a meal and can become aware of your learning or service development needs at these times. This is when you realise that other people are doing things differently from you and if they seem to be doing it better and achieving more, you can challenge yourself to decide if this matter could be one of your blind spots. Note down your thoughts before you forget them so that you can reflect on them later.

Online discussion groups may provide another source of informal exchanges with colleagues. If you find this difficult to start with, you might 'lurk', viewing the comments and views of other people until you feel confident enough to contribute. Record any observations that you find useful and reflect on how they might inform your own practice.

Observe your work environment and role

Observation could be informal and opportunistic, or more systematic working through a structured checklist. One method of self-assessment might be to audiotape yourself at work dealing with patients (after obtaining patients' informed consent). Listen to the tape afterwards to appraise your communication and consultation skills – on your own or with a friend or colleague. If you have access to video equipment, you might use this instead.

Look at the equipment in your workplace. Do you know how to operate it properly? Assess yourself undertaking practical procedures or ask someone to watch you operate the equipment or undertaking the practical procedure and give you feedback about your performance.

Analyse the various roles and responsibilities of your current posts. Compare your level of expertise against national standards such as in the Knowledge and Skills Framework for England from the Department of Health or a job evaluation framework as part of the Agenda for Change initiative.[19,20] Determine whether you can meet the requirements, or, if not, what deficiencies need to be made good.

You might combine one of the methods of identifying your learning needs already described such as an audit or SWOT analysis and apply it to 'observing your work environment or role', describing your relationship with other members of the multidisciplinary team for example, or reviewing how their roles and responsibilities interface with yours.

Read and reflect

When reading articles in respected journals, reflect on what the key messages mean for you in your situation. Note down topics about which you know little but that are relevant to your work and calculate if you have further learning needs not met by the article you are reading. If the article is relevant to your work, record what changes you will make and how you will make the changes. Record how you will impart your new knowledge to others in your workplace.

Educational review

You might find a buddy or work colleague, CPD tutor, or a clinical tutor or clinical supervisor with whom you can have an informal or formal discussion about your performance, job situation and learning needs. You might draw up a learning contract as a result with a timed plan of action.

Stage 3B: Identify your service needs – how you can find out if there are gaps in services or how you deliver care

Now focus your attention on the needs of your department or the trust. The standards of service delivery should be those that allow you to practise as a competent clinician. You may be competent but be unable to perform or practise to a competent level if the resources available to you are inadequate, or other colleagues have insufficient knowledge or skills to support you. You cannot be expected to take responsibility for ensuring that resources you need to be able to practise in a competent manner are available. However, as a professional you should play a significant role in collecting evidence to make a case for the need for essential resources to your colleagues, the manager, staff at the trust or primary care organisation (PCO) or whoever is appropriate.

Some of the methods you might use are described below and include:

- involving patients and the public in giving you feedback about the quality and quantity of your services
- monitoring access and availability to care
- undertaking a force-field analysis
- assessing risk
- evaluating the standards of care or services you provide
- comparing the systems in your practice with those required by legislation
- considering your patient population's health needs
- reviewing teamwork
- assessing the quality of your services
- reflecting on whether you are providing cost-effective care and services.

Involve patients and the public in giving you feedback about the quality and quantity of your services

Patient and public involvement may occur at three levels:

1 for individual patients about their own care
2 for patients and the public about the range and quality of health services on offer
3 in planning and organising health service developments.

The phrase 'patient and public involvement' is used here to mean individual involvement as a user, patient or carer, or public involvement that includes the processes of consultation and participation.[21]

If a patient involvement or public consultation exercise is to be meaningful, it has to involve people who represent the section of the population that the exercise is about. You will have to set up systems to actively seek out and involve people from minority groups or those with sensory impairments such as blind and deaf people.

Before you start:

- define the purpose
- be realistic about the magnitude of the planned exercise
- select an appropriate method or several methods depending on the target population and your resources
- obtain the commitment of everyone who will be affected by the exercise

- frame the method in accordance with your perspective
- write the protocol.

You might hold focus groups, or set up a patient panel, or invite feedback and help from a patient participation group. You could interview patients selected either at random from the patient population or for their experience of a particular condition or circumstance.

Monitor access to and availability of healthcare

You could look at waiting times to see a health professional by using:

- computerised appointment lists or paper and pen to record the time of arrival, the time of the appointment, the time seen
- the next available appointments that can easily be monitored by computer, or more painfully by manual searches of the appointment books.

Compare the results at intervals (a spreadsheet is a good way to do this). Do you or your staff have learning needs in relation to the use of technology, or new ways of redesigning the service you offer?

Referrals to other agencies and hospitals

You might audit and re-audit the time taken from the date the patient is seen to:

- the referral being sent (do you need more secretarial time?)
- the date the patient is seen by the other agency (could the patient be seen elsewhere quicker or do you need to liaise with other agencies over referrals?)
- the date the patient's needs have been met by investigation, diagnosis, treatment, provision of aid or support, etc (can you influence how quickly these are completed?).

Identify any learning needs here. For instance, new methods of teamwork with a different mix of skills between doctors, nurses and non-clinically qualified assistants could provide extra services in the department, or you, or a colleague, might retrain to provide a special clinical service.

Draw up a force-field analysis

This tool will help you to identify and focus down on the positive and negative forces in your work and to gain an overview of the weighting of these factors. Draw a horizontal or vertical line in the middle of a sheet of paper. Label one side 'positive' and the other side 'negative'. Draw bars to represent individual positive drivers that motivate you on one side of the line, and factors that are demotivating on the other negative side of the line. The thickness and length of the bars should represent the extent of the influence; that is, a short, narrow bar will indicate that the positive or negative factor has a minor influence and a long, wide bar a major effect. *See* Box 3.5 for an example.

Box 3.5: Example of force-field analysis diagram. Satisfaction with current post as a health professional

Positive factors (driving forces)	Negative factors (restraining forces)
career aspirations	long hours of work
salary	demands from patients
autonomy	
satisfaction from caring	job insecurity
no uniform	oppressive hierarchy
opportunities for professional development	

Take an overview of the resulting force-field diagram and consider if you are content with things as they are, or can think of ways to boost the positive side and minimise the negative factors. You can do this part of the exercise on your own, with a peer or a small group in the practice, or with a mentor or someone from outside the workplace. The exercise should help you to realise the extent to which a known influence in your life, or in the practice as a whole, is a positive or negative factor. Make a personal or organisational action plan to create the situations and opportunities to boost the positive factors in your life and minimise the bars on the negative side.

Assess risk

Risk assessment might entail evaluating the risks to the health or wellbeing or competence of yourself, staff and/or patients in your practice or workplace, and deciding on the action needed to minimise or eliminate those risks.[22] Risk assessment is part of the clinical governance framework of your organisation, which should have a standard process for reporting and reviewing adverse incidents, which may alert you to hazards through a root cause analysis where you aim to identify the fundamental cause(s) of the adverse event.

- *A hazard*: something with the potential to cause harm.
- *A risk*: the likelihood of that potential to cause harm being realised.

There are five steps to risk assessment:

1 look for and list the hazards
2 decide who might be harmed and how
3 evaluate the risks arising from the hazards and decide whether existing precautions are adequate or more should be done
4 record the findings
5 review your assessment from time to time and revise it if necessary.

You do not want to spend a lot of time and effort identifying risks or making changes if they do not matter much. When you have identified a risk, consider:

- is the risk large?
- does it happen often?
- is it a significant risk?

Risks may be prevented, avoided, minimised or managed where they cannot be eliminated. You, your colleagues and your staff may need to learn how to do this.

Record significant events where someone has experienced an adverse event or had a near miss – as part of you identifying your service development needs on an ongoing basis. Most significant incidents do not have one cause. Usually there are faults in the system, which are compounded by someone or several people being careless, tired, overworked or ill-informed. Cultivate an atmosphere of openness and discussion without blame so that you can all learn from the significant event. If people think they will be blamed they will hide the incident and no one will be able to prevent it happening again. Look for *all* the causes and try to remedy as many as possible to prevent the situation from arising in the future.

Evaluate the standards of services or care you provide

Keep your evaluation as simple as possible. Avoid wasting resources on unnecessarily bureaucratic evaluation. Design the evaluation so that you:

- specify the event (such as a service) to be evaluated – define broad issues, set priorities against strategic goals, time and resources, seek agreement on the nature and scope of the task
- describe the expected impact of the programme or activity and who will be affected
- define the criteria of success – these might relate to structure, process or outcome
- identify the information required to demonstrate the achievements of the programme or activity. The record might include: observing behaviour; data from existing records; prospective recording by the subjects of the programme or by the recipients and staff of the activity
- determine the time frame for the evaluation
- specify who collects the data for all stages in the delivery of the programme or activity, and the respective deadlines
- review and refine the objectives of the programme or activity and check that they are appropriate for the outcomes and impact you expect.

What to evaluate?

You could:

- adopt any, or all, of the six aspects of the health service's performance assessment framework: health improvement, fair access, effective delivery, efficiency, patient/carer experience, health outcomes
- agree milestones and goals at stages in your programme or adopt others such as relate to the National Service Frameworks
- evaluate the extent to which you achieve the outcome(s) starting with an objective. Alternatively, you might evaluate how conducive is the context of the programme, or activity, to achieving the anticipated outcomes
- undertake regular audits of aspects of the structure, process and outcome of a service or project to see if you have achieved what you expected when you established the criteria and standards of the audit programme
- evaluate the various components of a new system or programme: the activities, personnel involved, provision of services, organisational structure, precise goals and interventions.

Computer search

The extent to which you can evaluate your practice will depend on the quality of your records and extent to which you use the capacity of the computer at work. Compare the results of a computerised search for all those using one type of treatment with another in a practice. Make appropriate changes to your systems depending on what the computer search reveals. Put your plan into action and monitor with repeat searches at regular intervals.

Look at your learning or service development needs by analysing data from your records to:

- look at trends and patterns of illness
- devise and use clinical guidelines and decision support systems as part of evidence-based practice
- audit what you are doing
- provide the information on which to base decisions on commissioning and management
- support epidemiology, research and teaching activities.

Compare the systems in your department and practice with those required by legislation

Legislation changes quite frequently. You could start by comparing the systems at work with those required by the Disability Discrimination Act (1995)[23] and Health and Safety legislation.

Consider your patient population's health needs

Create a detailed profile of the population that you serve. Ask your public health lead for information about your patients and comparative information about the general population living in the district – morbidity and mortality statistics, referral patterns, age/sex mix, ethnicity, and population trends.

Include information about the wider determinants of health such as housing, numbers of the population in, and types of, employment, geographical location, the environment, crime and safety, educational attainment and socio-economic data. Make a note of any particular health problems such as higher than average teenage pregnancy rates or drug misuse. Focus on the current state of health inequalities within the patients you see or between them and the district as a whole. It may be that circumstances change, which in turn alters the proportion of minority groups in the population you serve – such as if there is an influx of homeless people or asylum seekers into your locality.

Review teamwork

You can measure how effective the team is[24] – evaluate whether the team has:

- clear goals and objectives
- accountability and authority
- individual roles for members
- shared tasks
- regular internal formal and informal communication
- full participation by members
- confrontation of conflict
- feedback to individuals
- feedback about team performance
- outside recognition
- two-way external communication
- team rewards.

Assess the quality of your services

Quality may be subdivided into eight components: equity, access, acceptability and responsiveness, appropriateness, communication, continuity, effectiveness and efficiency.[25]

You might use the matrix in Box 3.6 as a way of ordering your approach to auditing a particular topic with the eight aspects of quality on the vertical axis and structure, process and outcome on the horizontal axis.[26] In this way you can generate up to 24 aspects of a particular topic. You might then focus on several aspects to look at the quality of patient care or services from various angles.

Box 3.6:   Matrix for assessing the quality of a clinical service

You might look at the structure, process or outcome of communicating test results to patients for example.

	Structure	Process	Outcome
Equity			
Access			
Acceptability and responsiveness			
Appropriateness			
Communication	Hospital report	Feedback	Action taken
Continuity			
Effectiveness			
Efficiency			

Look for service development needs reflecting why patients receive a poor quality of service such as:

- inadequately trained staff or staff with poor levels of competence
- lack of confidentiality
- staff not being trained in the management of emergency situations
- doctors or nurses not being contactable in an emergency or being ineffective
- treatment being unavailable due to poor management of resources or services
- poor management of the arrangements for home visiting
- insufficient numbers of available staff for the workload
- qualifications of locums or deputising staff being unknown or inadequate for the posts they are filling
- arrangements for transfer of information from one team member to another being inadequate
- team members not acting on information received.

Many of these items will need action as a team, but for some of them, it may be your responsibility to ensure that adequate standards are met.

Reflect on whether you are providing cost-effective care and services

Cost-effectiveness is not synonymous with 'cheap'. A cost-effective intervention is one which gives a better or equivalent benefit from the intervention in question for lower or equivalent cost, or where the relative improvement in outcome is higher than the relative difference in cost. In other words being cost-effective means having the best outcomes for the least input. Using the term 'cost-effective' implies that you have considered potential alternatives.

An intervention must first be considered *clinically* effective to warrant investigation into its potential to be *cost*-effective. Evidence-based practice must incorporate clinical judgement. You have to interpret the evidence when it comes to applying it to individual patients, whether it is evidence about clinical effectiveness or cost-effectiveness. A new or alternative treatment or intervention should be compared directly with the previous best treatment or intervention.

An economic evaluation is a comparative analysis of two or more alternatives in terms of their costs and consequences. There are four different types as shown in Box 3.7.

Box 3.7:   The four types of economic evaluation

1   *Cost-effectiveness analysis* is used to compare the effectiveness of two inter-
     ventions with the same treatment objectives.
2   *Cost minimisation* compares the costs of alternative treatments that have
     identical health outcomes.
3   *Cost–utility analysis* enables the effects of alternative interventions to be
     measured against a combination of life expectancy and quality of life; common
     outcome measures are quality adjusted life years (QALYs) or health-related
     quality of life (hrqol).
4   *Cost–benefit analysis* is a technique designed to determine the feasibility of a
     project, plan, management or treatment by quantifying its costs and bene-
     fits. It is often difficult to determine these accurately in relation to health.

While health valuation is unavoidable, it cannot be objective. You will probably
have learning needs around what subjective method is best to use.[27]

Efficiency is sometimes confused with effectiveness. Being efficient means
obtaining the most quality from the least expenditure, or the required level of
quality for the least expenditure. To measure efficiency you need to make a
judgement about the level of quality of the 'purchase' and be able to relate it to
'price'. 'Price' alone does not measure efficiency. Quality is the indicator used
in combination with price to assess if something is more efficient. So, cost-
effectiveness is a measure of efficiency and suggests that costs have been
related to effectiveness.

Consider if you have service development needs. Discuss whether:

- the current skill mix in your team is appropriate
- more cost-effective alternative types of delivery of care are available
- sufficient staff training exists for those taking on new roles and responsibilities.

Set priorities: how you match what's needed with what's possible

You and your colleagues will have been able to make a wish list after following
the previous Stages 3A and 3B undertaking a variety of needs assessments.
Group and summarise your learning and service development needs from the
exercises you have carried out. Grade them according to the priority you set.
You may put one at a higher priority because it fits in with learning needs
established from another section, or put another lower because it does not fit in

with other activities that you will put into your learning plan for the next 12 months. If you have identified a learning need by several different methods of assessment then it will have a higher priority than something only identified once in your PDP. Collect information from all the team, the patients, users and carers to feed back before you make a decision on how to progress. Remember to take external influences into account such as the National Service Frameworks, NICE guidance, governmental priorities, priorities of your PCO, the content of the Local Delivery Plan, etc.

Select those topics that are tied into organisational priorities, have clear aims and objectives and are achievable within your time and resource constraints. When ranking topics for learning or action in order of priority (Stage 4) consider whether:

- the project aims and objectives are clearly defined
- the topic is important:
  - for the population served (e.g. the size of the problem and/or its severity)
  - for the skills, knowledge or attitudes of the individual or team
- it is feasible
- it is affordable
- it will make enough difference
- it fits in with other priorities.

You will still have more ideas than can possibly be implemented. Remember the highest priority – the health service is for patients that use it or who will do so in the future.

References

1 Rogers A (1986) *Teaching Adults*. Open University Press, Milton Keynes.

2 Schön DA (1987) *Educating the Reflecting Practitioner*. Jossey-Bass Publishers, San Francisco.

3 Rowntree D (1990) *Teaching through Self-instruction*. Kogan Page, London.

4 Wakley G, Cunnion M and Chambers R (2003) *Improving Sexual Health Advice*. Radcliffe Medical Press, Oxford.

5 Medical Professionalism Project (2002) Medical professionalism in the new millennium: a physicians' charter. *Lancet.* **359:** 520–2.

6 NHS Modernisation Agency website for PwSIs. www.gpwsi.org/subindex.shtml

7 Eraut M and du Boulay B (2000) *Developing the Attributes of Medical Professional Judgement and Competence*. University of Sussex, Sussex. Reproduced at www.informatics.sussex.ac.uk/users/bend/doh

8 Fraser SW and Greenhalgh T (2001) Coping with complexity: educating for capability. *British Medical Journal.* **323:** 799–802.

9 General Medical Council (2001) *Good Medical Practice.* General Medical Council, London.

10 Pendleton D, Schofield T, Tate P and Havelock P (2003) *The New Consultation, Developing Doctor–Patient Communication.* Oxford University Press, Oxford.

11 King J (2002) Career focus: 360° appraisal. *British Medical Journal.* **324:** S195.

12 Royal College of General Practitioners/General Practitioners Committee (2002) *Good Medical Practice for General Practitioners.* Royal College of General Practitioners, London.

13 National Institute for Clinical Excellence (NICE). www.nice.org.uk

14 Scottish Intercollegiate Guidelines Network (SIGN). www.sign.ac.uk

15 Royal College of Obstetricians and Gynaecologists website. www.rcog.org.uk

16 Irvine D and Irvine S (eds) (1991) *Making Sense of Audit.* Radcliffe Medical Press, Oxford.

17 Client-Focused Evaluations Program (CFEP). www.ex.ac.uk/cfep

18 Department of Health (2003) EPP Update newsletter. Department of Health, London. See Expert Patient Programme on www.ohn.gov.uk/ohn/people/expert.htm

19 Department of Health (2003) *The NHS Knowledge and Skills Framework (NHS KSF) and Development Review Guidance – working draft.* Version 6. Department of Health, London.

20 Department of Health (2003) *Job Evaluation Handbook.* Version 1. Department of Health, London.

21 Chambers R, Drinkwater C and Boath E (2003) *Involving Patients and the Public: how to do it better* (2e). Radcliffe Medical Press, Oxford.

22 Mohanna K and Chambers R (2000) *Risk Matters in Healthcare.* Radcliffe Medical Press, Oxford.

23 Disability Discrimination Act (1995) http://www.legislation.hmso.gov.uk/acts1995/1995050.htm
BBC Watchdog guide to Disability Discrimination Act http://www.bbc.co.uk/watchdog/guides_to/disability/

24 Hart E and Fletcher J (1999) Learning how to change: a selective analysis of literature and experience of how teams learn and organisations change. *Journal of Interprofessional Care.* **13(1):** 53–63.

25 Maxwell RJ (1984) Quality assessment in health. *British Medical Journal.* **288:** 1470–2.

26 Firth-Cozens J (1993) *Audit in Mental Health Services.* LEA, Hove.

27 McCulloch D (2003) *Valuing Health in Practice.* Ashgate Publishing Ltd, Aldershot.

4

Frameworks for training

This chapter considers various key professional reproductive health awards and frameworks for training. Areas covered include training at various levels of specialisation in both primary care and secondary care. Specific issues are presented regarding trainees coming from overseas to the UK and doctors opting for flexible working. A few of the learning resources with clear frameworks are mentioned, as are options for continuing professional development (CPD). The chapter concludes by drawing attention to the dynamic state of postgraduate education in the UK and the changes that may follow the 'Modernising Medical Careers' reforms.[1]

Diploma of the Royal College of Obstetricians and Gynaecologists (DRCOG)

The DRCOG is aimed at family practitioners who wish to provide an obstetric and gynaecological service within primary care. This qualification requires full registration with the GMC or Medical Council of Ireland, and by the time of registration completion of six consecutive months in a post recognised by the RCOG for the diploma examination. The examination comprises a multiple choice questionnaire and an objective, structured, clinical examination (OSCE). Further details of the exam including the syllabus are available at: www. rcog.org.uk/mainpages.asp?PageID=62.

Practitioners with special interests (PwSIs)

The NHS plans for England, Scotland, Wales and Northern Ireland identified the need to create new roles for GPs, nurses and allied professionals called 'practitioners with special clinical interests' (PwSIs).[2] A PwSI will be expected to act at an interim level of expertise, support and advice for local colleagues within the PCO.[3] This interim level of expertise is between that expected from an ordinary GP, nurse or allied professional carrying out their everyday work and that of a specialist with expertise derived from higher training. The Department of Health commissioned the RCGP to make recommendations for GPwSIs and specific recommendations for certain posts have now been made.[4] An example is given in Box 4.1.

Box 4.1:   Practitioner with a special interest (PwSI) in women's health

Two GPs who have had considerable experience and extra training run a referral clinic for their PCO, with back-up from the secondary care in the hospital trust. They do the initial management and investigation for patients with irregular or excessive menstrual loss, advise and fit long-term contraception (implants and intrauterine devices), manage problems with contraception such as patients with complex medical needs or difficulties with the contraception itself (lost intrauterine threads, etc) and run the pregnancy advice clinic.

Recommendations for nurses and practitioners allied to medicine are posted on the Department of Health website and will be updated as the posts evolve.[2] An example of one that is already working is given in Box 4.2.

Box 4.2:   Sexual health development nurse working as a PwSI

The sexual health development nurse at Guy's and St Thomas' Hospital Trust works across primary care and genitourinary (GU) medicine. Her work enables patients to be seen more quickly so that access is significantly improved. She acts as first point of contact for patients and has good links with bacteriologists, GPs and GU consultants.

Most health professionals have a special interest in one area or another. You may be involved in education, perhaps as a tutor or trainer; some of you may have a lead role within your PCO and others may do sessions in local family planning services and within other community or acute trust settings. A PwSI would be expected to provide an extended service, usually outside the confines of their practice and act independently. Different models of provision will be developed according to local need. Clinical accountability rests with the health professional who is responsible for his or her actions, including referral to specialist care and the need to work with other professional groups where appropriate. Overall accountability rests with the employing or contracting authority, usually a PCO. As a PwSI you would usually work with related acute trust services, with whom you may share premises, clinical governance activities, and participate in joint organisation and professional development when appropriate. A PwSI should be seen as one option available to the PCO for service delivery. This must be part of a co-ordinated approach to treatment services and not merely as a pragmatic solution to dealing with waiting lists. It is important that PwSIs are not seen as a substitute to a specialist service. Where a specialist provider is not in place then the PCO must ensure that a suitably trained practitioner fills this gap, rather than using the PwSI as a substitute.[4]

A health practitioner with a special interest in sexual health or women's health services would advise the PCO on the commissioning of care for these services.[5] You will need a health needs assessment to inform this process and you should be familiar with the process of health needs assessment for sexual health, contraceptive or women's health services.[6] Useful recommendations for the provision of contraceptive services, sexual health services and locally enhanced services appear on the website of the Faculty of Family Planning and Reproductive Health Care.[7]

The following are examples of core activities of a PwSI service:[3,4]

- clinical services provided in general practice premises, community or acute trust clinics, and outreach venues, such as youth clubs, hostels or domiciliary services. These might include:
  - advice on, and provision for, contraception for people with complex medical or social problems
  - provision of long-acting methods of contraception including sterilisation
  - abortion counselling and services
  - investigation and treatment of abnormal vaginal bleeding
  - management of menopausal problems
  - advice, investigation and treatment of sexually transmitted infections
- education and liaison, in partnership with others, to provide:
  - support, facilities and expertise for the development of training for health professionals
  - information and support to practices and practitioners on best practice
  - a bridge between primary and specialist women's health services
- leadership to:
  - develop pathways of care for patients, including the development of local referral and treatment guidance
  - develop clinical capacity for patients in primary care either as part of local or nationally enhanced services, as defined in the new GMS contract
  - support the development of risk management and harm reduction across the PCO.

This is a rapidly evolving field. Recommendations and regulations are likely to change, so you will need to keep abreast of what is expected of you at this level of expertise and competence. Membership of the Faculty of Family Planning and Reproductive Health Care or an MSc in Community Gynaecology and

Reproductive Health Care could be suitable starting points from which to demonstrate your level of competence.[7,8]

Membership of the Royal College of Obstetricians and Gynaecologists (MRCOG)

The MRCOG is intended for those who wish to specialise in obstetrics and gynaecology. The exam is taken in two parts. The first part may be taken any time after gaining a medical degree, whereas the second part may only be taken after a period of appropriate training as detailed at the web address below. Part 1 MRCOG examination covers basic sciences and consists of two multiple choice question papers. Part 2 MRCOG examination starts with an MCQ paper and written papers. Only those candidates who achieve a minimum standard proceed to the remainder of the examination, which consists of a three-hour oral assessment divided into a sequence of 12 stations each lasting 15 minutes. Individual stations are diverse in nature testing factual knowledge and understanding, problem-solving skills, diagnosis, investigation, treatment, clinical skills and communication skills. Further details are available at: www. rcog.org.uk/mainpages.asp?PageID=61.

Structured training resources aimed at trainees in obstetrics and gynaecology (StratOG)

As part of its support for specialist training, the RCOG has produced StratOG, which is a comprehensive distance learning programme. StratOG provides a framework for learning using a syllabus that fits in with day-to-day activity giving clear objectives to help pass the Part 2 MRCOG (or equivalent) examination. Essentially StratOG comprises 10 paper-based study modules including interactive tutorials and a supporting website with various relevant resources and interactive forum. Further details are available at: www.rcog. org.uk/mainpages.asp?PageID=98.

Obstetrics and Gynaecology Certificate of Completion of Specialist Training (CCST)

Although there are a number of types of specialist registrars, only specialist registrars in a type 1 programme holding a national training number (NTN) may complete a higher specialist programme and achieve a CCST (*see* Box 4.3). Possession of the CCST entitles the holder to be entered on the Specialist Register of the General Medical Council hence being eligible to become a substantive consultant in the UK. Entry to a type 1 training post is in open competition amongst trainees who have completed two years of basic specialist training, at least one year in clinical obstetrics and gynaecology and passed the Part 1 MRCOG.

The RCOG oversees the quality of training, setting standards and ultimately is responsible to the Specialist Training Authority (STA) for recommending the award of the CCST. Specific specialist registrar training posts are managed by the deaneries ensuring generic requirements are met (*see* Box 4.4). The management of the training programmes is carried out by the deanery specialist training committees, which include junior doctor representation. Higher training is divided into core specialist training (Years 1–3), by the end of which the Part 2 MRCOG should be passed, and advanced specialist training (Years 4–5).

Trainees must complete satisfactory annual assessment through a record of in-training assessment (RITA) interview by a small panel, which includes the specialist training committee (STC) chairman or specialty adviser, and training programme directors. At interview the progress of the trainee is assessed by information received from local assessment including logbooks to decide whether the trainee can proceed to the next year of training or whether the trainee needs specially focused training, possibly being held back. Appeals may be made if a trainee disagrees with a decision for focused training or delay to the CCST date. Following completion of core specialist training, trainees may seek special interest or subspecialist training (*see* page 66). There are seven forms available for the RITA process and if at the end of the training programme a satisfactory RITA G is given, a CCST is awarded (*see* Box 4.5). Further details are available at: www.rcog.org.uk/mainpages.asp?PageID=93.

Box 4.3:   Specialist register training grades

Type 1 programme
The training grade leading to award of CCST. UK trainees hold a national training number (NTN) whereas overseas doctors hold a visiting training number (VTN) (*see* text).

Type 2 programme or fixed term training appointment (FTTA)
This training grade provides an opportunity for overseas doctors, who hold a fixed term training number (FTN) (*see* text).

LAT (locum appointment for training)
This may last from three months to a year, but must be recognised prospectively by the RCOG. They are similar to a FTTA except they carry educational credit, which may count towards a CCST if the holder subsequently gains a type 1 appointment.

LAS (locum appointment for service)
This may last up to three months but does not carry educational credit.

With the above training posts it is possible to apply for a flexible training scheme hence working between 50% and 80% of a standard working week, if there are 'well-founded' reasons for being unable to train full time. Trainees have to show that training on a full-time basis would not be practical in view of, for instance, domestic commitments, disability or ill-health. Domestic commitments are normally understood to mean caring for another e.g. child or an elderly relative rather than just being married/having a partner. For further information *see*: www.rcog.org.uk/mainpages.asp?PageID=660.

Box 4.4:   Ten requirements for specialist registrar training posts in the West Midlands Deanery

1   *Programme director*: each specialty training specialist registrar must have a named programme director who accepts responsibility with the clinical tutor for planning the programme and ensuring that the standards set out below are met within the specialty.

2   *Protected teaching*: at least 3 h of protected teaching, based on the Royal College or Faculty curriculum, and separate from clinical work, must be provided weekly. Specialist registrars must attend a minimum of 70% of these. The programme must be evaluated by the trainees and modified in the light of discussion and feedback obtained.

3   *Educational supervision*: every specialist registrar must have a named educational supervisor, who meets with the specialist registrar privately at the start of each attachment, and then three monthly for appraisal, to clarify career goals, identify learning needs and plan the education accordingly. Information from the consultant trainer (if different) about the specialist registrar's progress must be provided for these sessions.

4   *Feedback/appraisal/assessment*: all consultants involved in supervising specialist registrars must provide regular informal constructive feedback on both good and poor performance and contribute to appraisal and assessment of the specialist registrar.

5   *Induction*: at the beginning of each post, all specialist registrars must attend induction programmes designed to familiarise them with the trust in general

and the specialty department in which they will be working (in terms of both organisational and educational aspects). Written information on timetables, guidelines and other arrangements must be provided.

6 *Audit/clinical guidelines/research*: written guidelines on the management of common clinical conditions agreed by all consultants in the specialty must be available to the specialist registrar. These should be evidence based and subject to audit. Specialist registrars must be actively involved personally in audit. Time for research where appropriate and agreed in advance must be made available.

7 *Senior doctor cover*: the immediate availability of advice from a consultant must be available to specialist registrars. In line with Royal College guidelines, according to specialty, each specialist registrar must attend at least two consultant-led ward rounds, two outpatient clinics and two consultant-led operating sessions (for surgical specialties) per week.

8 *Clinical activity*: all specialist registrars must be exposed to a level of clinical activity appropriate to their stage of educational development, for the achievement of their educational objectives.

9 *Inappropriate tasks*: no specialist registrar should be exposed to work for which they are inadequately trained, or work of no relevance to their educational objectives, including working in more junior roles.

10 *Study leave*: specialist registrars must be allowed to attend courses appropriate to their educational objectives, agreed in advance with their educational supervisor, within their educational plan, and within the limits set by the postgraduate dean.

Box 4.5: Forms available for the RITA process

- *Form A*: core information on the trainee, issued on appointment and, once signed by the trainee and training programme director/STC chairman, sent to college to register the start of training
- *Form B*: used to record changes in core information
- *Form C*: record of satisfactory progress within the specialist registrar grade
- *Form D*: recommendation for targeted training – stage 1 of 'required additional training'
- *Form E*: recommendation for intensified supervision/repeated experience – stage 2 of 'required additional training'
- *Form F*: record of out-of-programme experience allowing flexibility for trainees to acquire experience outside the programme but complementary to it
- *Form G*: final record of satisfactory progress

Royal College of Obstetricians and Gynaecologists special interest training

In 1999, a RCOG working party proposed 'special skills training' defined as 'specific skills that are beyond those required for the acquisition of a CCST in clinical, teaching and managerial aspects of obstetrics and gynaecology'.[9] The special interest skills are provided as a series of modules usually produced in partnership with specialist professional bodies (*see* Table 4.1). It is intended these modules are taken in specialist registrar (SpR) Years 4 and 5 during the one and/or probably two sessions a week dedicated to private study. Usually a module should be completed within one year thus trainees may be able to complete two modules prior to obtaining their CCST. Further details are available at: www.rcog.org.uk/mainpages.asp?PageID=1041.

Table 4.1:   RCOG special interest training modules 2004

Module	Specialist society
Assisted reproduction	British Fertility Society
Management of the infertile couple	British Fertility Society
Maternal medicine	British Maternal and Fetal Medicine Society
Menopause	British Menopause Society
Obstetric leadership on the labour ward	British Maternal and Fetal Medicine Society
Ultrasound imaging in the management of gynaecological conditions Urodynamics	British Society of Urogynaecology

Royal College of Obstetricians and Gynaecologists subspecialty training

Subspecialty training is an extensive highly intensive advanced specialist training in a single subspecialty (*see* Box 4.6). Obstetricians and gynaecologists, who successfully complete this additional higher training, are recognised to have special expertise and experience in the relevant field. The training programmes are for three years, although trainees may gain exemptions for part of a programme if they have completed appropriate research or clinical experience. Further details are available at: www.rcog.org.uk/mainpages.asp?PageID=84.

> **Box 4.6:**   RCOG subspecialty training programmes
> - Gynaecological oncology
> - Maternal and fetal medicine
> - Reproductive medicine
> - Sexual and reproductive health
> - Urogynaecology

Genitourinary Medicine Certificate of Completion of Specialist Training (CCST)

The Royal College of Physicians oversees higher medical training in GUM, outlining a syllabus that includes gynaecology, family planning, dermatology, infectious diseases, public health medicine and laboratory work such as microbiology, virology and forensic microbiology. Applicants should have completed a minimum of two years' general professional training (GPT) in approved posts and obtained the MRCP (UK) or (I), or MRCOG. Holders of the MRCP must obtain appropriate gynaecological experience at some stage of their training, whereas MRCOG entrants must have spent at least 12 months in posts providing some general medical experience before they can be appointed. The higher medical training programme lasts four years. Further details are available at: www.rcplondon.ac.uk.

Doctors coming to train in the NHS from overseas

Overseas doctors may come to the UK for a variety of training opportunities including preparation for Royal College examinations. Often they take a post as senior house officers (SHOs) to prepare for examinations or gain the necessary basic specialist training in the UK to apply for specialist registrar posts. Foreign, non-UK graduate doctors, who are about to start their first post in the NHS, may take advantage of a free induction course to help their transition to working in this new environment. For further information telephone NHS Professionals on +44 (0)845 1203164.

Type 2 Specialist Training Programme or fixed term training appointment (FTTA)

The purpose of this appointment is to provide overseas doctors, without a right of indefinite residence, a modified training programme tailored, where feasible, to their personal goals. Usually this specialist registrar appointment is between 6 months and 24 months with a corresponding amount of permit-free training. Training does not attract educational credit thus it can not lead to the award of a CCST irrespective of duration. In order to progress to CCST an overseas doctor must be appointed to a type 1 programme in open competition. Once on a type 1 programme, the doctor may initially receive three years' permit-free training which can be extended to gain a CCST if necessary. However, possession of a CCST does not provide right of indefinite residence.

The RCOG co-ordinates an Overseas Training Fellowship Scheme providing salaried higher training for two years at the first stage of the specialist registrar grade. As with all trainees, continuation on the programme is conditional on satisfactory regular appraisal and the initial six months is a probation period. Eligibility criteria are given in Box 4.7 and further information is available at: www.rcog.org.uk/mainpages.asp?PageID=83.

Box 4.7:   Eligibility criteria for RCOG Overseas Training Fellowship Scheme

- Part 1 MRCOG (or equivalent by recognised exemption)
- International English Language Testing System (IELTS) academic module at the approved level (7.0 in all four components) with at least 12 months remaining at the time of application
- Three years of supervised postgraduate practice in obstetrics and gynaecology which has been approved by the examination department towards Part 2 MRCOG examination
- Have had training for the Part 2 MRCOG examination assessed by the examination department of the RCOG
- Be currently domiciled in their home country
- Not have been previously registered with the UK GMC

Continuing professional development (CPD)

CPD implies professional lifelong learning, which in medicine includes knowledge and skills both in the clinical specialty and in a doctor's wider role. Both consultant and non-consultant grade career staff working in any aspect of obstetrics and gynaecology must follow the RCOG UK CPD programme unless they notify the RCOG of alternative professional arrangements. In addition the RCOG provides an optional Overseas CPD Programme for fellows and members of the college who are in practice overseas. Further information is available at: www.rcog.org.uk/mainpages.asp?PageID=1441 (*see* Box 4.8).

Box 4.8: Outline of requirements for participation in the RCOG CPD programmes

The main distinction between the overseas and UK programmes relates to the location where local category activities are undertaken.

UK programme

- Requirement for participation: collection of at least 250 credits every five years.
- The programme framework is divided into two distinct areas of learning:
  - clinical educational activities directly relevant to the unique requirements of obstetricians and gynaecologists. This forms the core of the CPD programme with a required minimum of 50 credits in each of the three categories of activity: local, external and personal
  - non-clinical educational activities or clinical educational activities relating to the general skills and knowledge applicable to all doctors. No minimum requirement is laid down for this area of activity which comprises the professional category.
- CPD participants are required to record details of CPD activities in their CPD diary and to compile a CPD file comprising evidence of their activities.
- Participants must inform the CPD office of their progress annually and are required to return their diary for spot-checking at least once during the five-year cycle.
- Once registered on the programme, participants will be able to participate fully in the questions provided in *The Obstetrician & Gynaecologist* by returning their response form to the college for marking. The time allowed for completion of response forms is six months.
- Names of all participants who successfully complete their five-year cycle are published on the UK CPD Roll.[10]

Overseas programme

- Requirement for participation: collection of at least 250 credits every five years to include a minimum of 50 local category, 50 external category and 50 personal category credits.
- Participants are required to record details of CPD activities in their continuing medical education (CME) diary and to compile a CPD file comprising evidence of their activities.

- Participants must inform the CPD office of their progress annually and are required to return their diary for spot-checking at least once during the five-year cycle.
- Once registered on the programme, participants will be able to participate fully in the questions provided in *The Obstetrician & Gynaecologist* by returning their response form to the college for marking. The time allowed for completion of response forms is six months.
- Names of all participants who successfully complete their five-year cycle are published on the Overseas CPD Roll.[10]

Distance interactive learning in obstetrics and gynaecology (DIALOG)

As part of its educational support the RCOG has produced DIALOG, which is an interactive computer-based learning package delivered on CD ROM. Completion of tasks provides the career grade staff with RCOG CPD credits. Further DIALOG may help postgraduate trainees prepare for MRCOG, DRCOG and other postgraduate specialist qualifications. The computer-based learning includes interactive case studies relevant to current practice allowing the user to proceed at his/her pace with instant feedback. For further information *see*: www.rcog.org.uk/mainpages.asp?PageID=97.

Reproduction and Development MSc, diploma and certificate

The importance and demand for postgraduate medical education including CPD is growing rapidly both in the UK and worldwide. However, inflexible study frameworks of conventional university courses may not fit with people's career paths or lifestyles. One option is to offer flexible programmes using distance learning models that widen participation further by reducing geographical restrictions particularly when using the internet. Since 1995 the ReproMED project, based in the University of Bristol, has pioneered the use of the internet to support biomedical postgraduate education. Following a critical review of the place of information technology to support postgraduate education leading to a prize-winning website,[11,12] the ReproMED project ran a pilot training programme providing reproductive medicine education over the internet.[13] Following the success of the pilot programme in 2001 ReproMED launched a comprehensive training programme delivered over the internet covering

Reproduction and Development aimed at a multiprofessional international student group providing masters, diploma and certificate options of study.[14]

The Reproduction and Development MSc is a modular course that may be followed either full time, taking one year to complete, or part time taking two years to complete. Options are also provided at certificate and diploma levels for those who may not choose to complete the whole course or fail to complete all modules to the necessary standards. The course utilises distance learning methodology with the majority of teaching delivered over the internet. Students are only required to physically attend Bristol for around 10 weeks over their entire study period. The time spent in Bristol is arranged into twice yearly workshops – at the start of each academic year and six months later. The course is composed of six taught modules and a research dissertation. Each of the taught modules is allocated a week of workshop space and during this time students attend lectures, lab and clinically orientated practical sessions and computer workshops. Periods between workshops are structured with assessed coursework to ensure students cover the entire syllabus and spend time on their research project. Coursework takes the form of essays, short answers, computer assisted assessments, practical reports and online discussion forums. Students are supported through their home-study periods with tutor contact via email and telephone and a course website. The website provides a range of resources such as lectures, interactive tutorials, collaborative discussion forums, access to internet search engines and full text electronic journals together with administrative information about the programme. The programme has proven to be extremely popular and it is likely that this method of postgraduate education will increase greatly in the future. For further information *see*: www.red-msc.org.uk.

'Modernising Medical Careers'

It is important to be aware that UK postgraduate medical education is currently undergoing a major reform following a *Policy Statement on Modernising Medical Careers* published in February 2003 by the four UK Health Departments.[15,16] *The Policy Statement on Modernising Medical Careers* outlines seven principles underlying training: trainee centred, competency assessed, service based, quality assured, flexible, coached and structured, and streamlined. After a process of consultation in April 2004 a key document outlining details of change was published: *The Next Steps – the future shape of foundation, specialist and general practice training programmes*.[17] All medical school graduates will enter a two-year foundation programme to learn core clinical skills so they will be able to care for the acutely ill patient. In addition doctors will be expected to develop their communication, teamworking and IT skills.

The Joint Committee on Postgraduate Training for General Practice (JCPTGP) and the Specialist Training Authority (STA) are being replaced by the Post-graduate Medical Education and Training Board (PMETB) who will oversee the standards and quality of postgraduate medical education and training in the UK. This new board will review and set the standards and frameworks for current and new 'streamlined' training programmes utilising the experience and expertise of the medical Royal Colleges. The board will issue Certificates of Completion of Training (CCT) to doctors successfully completing training programmes replacing the current CCST. The board may also assess doctors trained overseas without UK-recognised qualifications to decide whether they may be registered or additional training and assessment is required. For further information *see*: www.mmc.nhs.uk.

References

1 www.mmc.nhs.uk

2 Visit Department of Health website and use the search facility for the most recent information. www.dh.gov.uk

3 Wakley G and Chambers R (2002) *Sexual Health Matters in Primary Care.* Radcliffe Medical Press, Oxford.

4 NHS Modernisation Agency step-by-step guide to setting up GPwSI services. www.gpwsi.org/stepbystep/

5 Department of Health (2003) *Effective Commissioning of Sexual Health and HIV Services – A sexual health and HIV commissioning toolkit for primary care trusts and local authorities.* Department of Health, London.

6 Wakley G, Cunnion M and Chambers R (2003) *Improving Sexual Health Advice.* Radcliffe Medical Press, Oxford.

7 Faculty of Family Planning and Reproductive Health Care. www.ffprhc.org.uk

8 University of Warwick. www.warwick.ac.uk/fac/sci/Medical

9 RCOG (1999) Working Party Report on Special Skills Training. October. www.rcog.org.uk/mainpages.asp?PageID=1041

10 www.rcog.org.uk/mainpages.asp?PageID=116

11 www.SWOT.org.uk

12 Draycott TJ, Cook J, Fox R and Jenkins J (1999) Information technology for postgraduate education: a survey of facilities and skills in the South West Deanery. *British Journal of Obstetrics and Gynaecology.* **106:** 731–5.

13 Jenkins J, Cook J, Edwards J, Draycott T and Cahill D (2001) A pilot Internet training programme in reproductive medicine. *British Journal of Obstetrics and Gynaecology.* **108:** 114–16.

14 Whittington K, Cook J, Barratt C and Jenkins J (2004) Can the Internet widen participation in reproductive medicine education for professionals? *Human Reproduction.* **19:** 1800–5.

15 Donaldson L (2002) *Unfinished Business – proposals for reform of the SHO grade.* www.mmc.nhs.uk/keyarticles/SHOREPORT.pdf

16 Four UK Health Departments (2003) *Policy Statement on Modernising Medical Careers.* www.mmc.nhs.uk/keyarticles/FINAL_VERSION_UK_POLICY_STA.pdf

17 Four UK Health Departments (2004) *The Next Steps – the future shape of foundation, specialist and general practice training programmes.* www.mmc.nhs.uk/keyarticles/NEXT_STEPS_FUTURE_FOUND-SPEC-GP.pdf

5

Contraception and termination of pregnancy

Contraception

Although most discussion of contraception will occur in primary care or in community clinics, a considerable number of women attend the gynaecology clinic for whom the choice of contraception is directly relevant to their gynaecological management, thus gynaecologists must understand contraception. Referral for consideration of sterilisation is a frequent request as it involves a surgical procedure usually under general anaesthesia.

Avoiding unwanted pregnancies is desirable for women, although each contraceptive method available has different risks and benefits. Side-effects or disadvantages perceived as significant for that woman or for the couple reduce compliance and lead to contraceptive failures. The level of teenage pregnancy and the proportion of pregnancies being terminated are both socially and politically important. Providing women with information about the benefits and possible risks of different contraceptive methods available will allow them to reach a decision on which method is most appropriate.

PwSIs in reproductive health will need excellent knowledge and skills in contraception. They should be capable of managing and supplying longer-acting methods of contraception. They should have expertise in advising on the special needs of women with medical conditions such as Crohn's disease or diabetes. Much of their work will involve the management of problems with or queries about contraception. They will usually demonstrate their competence by external examinations such as the Membership of the Faculty of Family Planning and/or an MSc in reproductive health (*see* Chapter 4).

Case study 5.1

Two young women attend together. Miss Giddy was referred with painful heavy periods and you have been able to tell her that she has no medical problem causing this. You offer treatment with non-steroidal anti-inflammatory drugs, or the option of going on the pill and they look at each other. Miss Brain explains that Miss Giddy wants to know if she can go on the pill without her GP knowing as she thinks her mother will then know. Miss Giddy's mother is 'against the pill' as she thinks Miss Giddy is too young to have intercourse. However, this is already occurring and Miss Brain is worried that Miss Giddy will get pregnant. They have talked it over and Miss Giddy now wants to go on the pill like Miss Brain.

What issues you should cover

Confidentiality

Explain that the doctors have a duty to keep her medical information confidential. That is, no one else needs to know unless there is a risk to her health or to someone else's health, which would mean that other people would need to know. It would always be discussed with her if confidential information needed to be passed to someone else. You would like to let her regular doctor know about the contraceptive consultation but only if she agrees. You have, of course, already given her the choice of being seen by herself or with her friend. Explain, too, that her mother may be happy to know that she is on the pill to control her periods. Whether she tells her mother that she is also using it as a contraceptive is up to her, but her mother might well be relieved as she may be worried about the possibility but not know how to bring the subject up.

Risk of pregnancy

Explain that you need to know a bit about her to find out if it is safe for her to start taking the contraceptive pill. First, establish if she is intending to continue to be sexually active. If she is, then you need to know if she is using any other method of contraception (e.g. condoms). Ask if, and when, she has had any unprotected sexual intercourse and the date of her last menstrual period, in case she needs emergency contraception or is already pregnant (*see* information on emergency contraception later in this chapter).

You could also explain that although lots of young people say that they are having sexual intercourse, confidential surveys have shown that eight out of ten young people under the age of 16 years have not actually started having sexual intercourse. It may be better for her to go on the pill just in case but she does not have to have sexual intercourse unless she wants to.

Age and the law

If she is living in the parental home, whatever her age, it is much simpler for her to have discussed her need for contraception at home so that there is no need for concealment. Discuss how she might do this, if she has not already done so. The younger the woman, the more important it is to establish whether this discussion has taken place and whether the woman herself understands the full implications of her actions. Keep in mind the Fraser Guidelines (*see* Box 5.1).[1]

Box 5.1:   The Fraser Guidelines[1]

The guidelines were drawn up after Lord Fraser stated in 1985 that a doctor could give contraceptive advice or treatment to a person under 16 years old without parental consent, providing that the doctor is satisfied that:

* the young person will understand the advice
* the young person cannot be persuaded to tell their parents or allow the doctor to tell them that they are seeking contraceptive advice
* the young person is likely to begin or continue having unprotected sex with or without contraceptive treatment
* the young person's physical or mental health is likely to suffer unless they receive contraceptive advice or treatment
* it is in the young person's best interest to give contraceptive advice or treatment.

The Fraser Guidelines apply to health professionals in England and Wales. In Scotland, the Age of Legal Capacity (Scotland) Act 1991 gives similar powers of consent to those under 16 years of age. In Northern Ireland, separate similar legislation applies.

The Fraser Guidelines are included within the best practice guidance for doctors and other health professionals on the provision of advice and treatment to young people under 16 on contraception, sexual and reproductive health published by the Department of Health in July 2004.[1]

Her plans for the future

Find out how important it is for her not to be pregnant. Young women may say that they are not bothered whether they get pregnant or not. This is often because they have no belief in their own ability to control their future – or because they do not have any vision of their future at all; things just happen to them. Talking to them about what they want to do in the future can help them to see when a pregnancy might be more easily managed.

It may be extremely important for the woman not to become pregnant. Women who have definite plans – for a job, for training or further education – are usually well motivated to use contraception. Some young women are definite (at least for the time being) that they never want children.

Reasons why she may not have used contraception

The Social Exclusion Unit report[2] attributes high rates of teenage conception in the UK to young people's:

- low expectations
- lack of knowledge about contraception and how it can be obtained
- lack of understanding about what is involved in forming relationships and parenting
- reception of mixed messages from society – 'it sometimes seems as if sex is compulsory but contraception is illegal' as one of the young people cited in the report said.[2]

In a national survey of 515 teenagers aged 12 to 17 years, more than half of the respondents said that the main reason young people do not use birth control was because of drinking alcohol or using drugs. Boys and girls gave similar answers. Half of the teenagers quizzed thought another common reason for young people having unprotected sex was pressure from partners who do not want to use contraception. Young adolescents aged 12 to 14 years were as likely as the older teenagers to say this.[3]

Problems associated with teenage pregnancy

The death rate for babies of teenage mothers is 60% higher than that for babies of older mothers, and maternal and fetal risks are highest in under-16 year olds.

Pregnant teenagers are more likely than mothers aged 20 to 35 years to have low income, poor education, be unwed, be cigarette smokers, and have poor nutrition. The Acheson report[4] on health inequalities recognised that teenage mothers and children are at higher risk of experiencing adverse health, educational, social and economic outcomes, compared to older mothers and their children.[4]

Teenage pregnancy is a cause and effect of inequalities in health. Teenage mothers tend to have poor antenatal care, low birthweight infants and higher infant mortality rates. Teenage parents tend to miss out on education and have substantially lower incomes. They are more likely to suffer from postnatal depression and relationship breakdown. Risk factors for teenage pregnancy include: having a teenage mother, divorced parents, deprivation, being a child living in care, educational problems, sexual abuse, ethnicity, mental health problems and crime.[3]

What she may know about contraception already

Some young women are well informed and have read many leaflets. Others know little or nothing. Make sure that you mention other methods of contraception apart from the pill that her friend has already suggested. Using a leaflet that summarises all the methods enables you to go through each method and its level of contraceptive protection quite rapidly, so that she can make her own choice for discussion in more detail.[5]

Check that she is safe to use her chosen contraceptive

Most young women will be healthy and have no contraindications to any method of contraception. For them, any method of contraception is preferable to the risks of pregnancy (although you can tell her that abstinence is the safest method of all, provided it does not fail!). You need to take a medical history to ensure that her chosen method will not do harm. Checking her blood pressure before giving contraceptives containing oestrogen is essential, but other physical examination is not necessary unless indicated by the history. Obesity and/or smoking increase her risks of venous thrombosis and cardiovascular disease. The absolute risk of venous thrombosis in a young woman is small, but lifestyle advice now may help her to make changes to avoid an increased risk in the future. However, keep in mind that she has come for contraceptive advice, not a lecture on her bad habits – or she will not want to return to see health professionals if she thinks she will have a lecture.

You may wish to use a checklist to exclude contraindications. The World Health Organization (WHO) publishes a checklist with advice on cautions and contraindications.[6] A UK adaptation of the WHO advice appears on the website for the Faculty of Family Planning and Reproductive Health Care.[7]

Summarising where the consultation has reached

The consultation has probably already lasted 10 minutes. You may need to summarise where you are and ask her what she wants to do next. If she has an urgent need for contraception (most young people do not attend until they do need it urgently), your next action is to take the extra time to help her learn how to use the method she has chosen. If she wants to use a long-acting method, she might be better using a short-acting method temporarily. Discuss how she could return to see an appropriate health professional later in a young people's clinic or at her GP's surgery. This gives her time to discuss the method in more depth and for a more considered decision on a method that she cannot change easily. (Long-acting methods are discussed later in this chapter in Table 5.1.)

She and her sexual partner should use condoms for protection against method failure (common when people first start using contraception) and against sexually transmitted infections (STIs). She should be clear that most people do not have any symptoms from STIs and that appearances are no guide as to whether someone is infected or not.

A young woman who is still living with her parents or guardians can be helped to realise that they may be worried about whether she is protected against pregnancy, but may be uncertain how to ask her if she is at risk. Talk about ways she might discuss this with them.

Using short-acting methods

CONDOMS

You need to know how she can obtain condoms. Discuss with her how she is going to ask her partner to use condoms, how she will carry condoms (many young people do not have handbags or pockets) and that the condom should be put on the penis after erection but before genital contact.

She can obtain free supplies from family planning clinics, sexual health clinics and youth clinics, such as Brook or locally developed services. You should know where the local suppliers are, when they are open, and how she can be seen (does she need an appointment or is it open access?). She can go with her sexual partner or he can obtain condoms from the same places himself, so that he can be sure how to use them correctly. She, or her partner, can buy condoms from many outlets, including vending machines, chemists, supermarkets and garages.

Female condoms (Femidom) need to be used carefully so that the penis is placed inside the polyurethane sleeve lining the vagina. They are rather expensive – but can be bought over the counter with no need for medical intervention. They are disliked by some people because of the 'plastic mac' feel and are noisy in use.

ORAL METHODS

She may decide to start on the combined oral contraceptive (COC) or the progestogen only pill (POP). It is useful to go through the leaflet with her that you will give her to take away.[5] This ensures that the advice you give and the advice in the leaflet is the same (or that you have handwritten any changes and explained the reasons for them). Tell her that the leaflet in the packet of pills may give slightly different advice depending on how long ago it was written.

Give her the choice of starting immediately or waiting for the first day of her next period. If she starts immediately, she should not rely on the pill for her contraception for the first seven days. If she starts on the first day of her menstrual cycle, she will be protected against pregnancy immediately, but will still need to use condoms for extra safety and protection against the risk of STIs.

Help her to decide what time of day will be easiest for her to remember to take her pill. Show her a packet of the pill she will be taking or a diagram in the leaflet of how to take the pill. Show her the section in the leaflet on what to do if she misses a pill, and go through the instructions as this is the commonest cause of failure. Advise her how to stop smoking if she is a cigarette smoker.

She should contact her GP or the practice nurse or community clinic (explain how) before her review appointment if she has any queries that are not explained in the leaflet, or new serious health complaints. Point out the types of condition, listed in the leaflet, that should take her to the doctor urgently (e.g. shortness of breath, leg pain and swelling, first or worsening migraine, or dizziness).

EMERGENCY CONTRACEPTION[7,8,9]

One of the reasons Miss Giddy may be asking about going on the pill now could be that she has had unprotected sexual intercourse and requires emergency contraception.

The oral emergency contraceptives Levonelle or Levonelle-2 can be used up to 72 h after unprotected intercourse, but the earlier the better. Levonelle and Levonelle-2 both contain the same doses of progestogen. Levonelle is the version bought over the counter and Levonelle-2 is the prescribed version. Levonelle is 95% effective in preventing pregnancy when taken within 24 h of unprotected sexual intercourse. It is 85% effective when taken 25–48 h later and only 58% effective when taken between 49 and 72 h later. New administration advice is for both pills to be taken together.

Increased doses of hormone are necessary for patients on hepatic enzyme inducers such as phenytoin, carbamezepine or rifampicin to obtain the same blood levels. Most guidelines advise two pills followed by either another one or two 12 h later.[7] Box 5.2 summarises the information you will need to elicit to decide whether oral emergency contraception should be prescribed and what advice to give. You could use this to draw up a protocol.

Box 5.2: Emergency contraception tablets: basic information required and advice

Minimum information to be recorded in the notes prior to prescribing oral post-coital contraception should include:

- last menstrual period (LMP)
- cycle length
- date and time of unprotected sexual intercourse (UPSI)
- day of cycle of UPSI

- any other UPSI since LMP
- options discussed (oral/intrauterine device (IUD))
- any interacting medication
- current liver disease.

Counselling should include:

- likelihood of nausea
- mode of action
- failure rate
- side-effects
- timing of next period
- action to take if next period is not on time
- discussion of future contraception needs.

Vomiting after taking emergency combined oral contraception
If the patient vomits within 2 h of taking the pills, she should be advised to seek further medical advice. Domperidone 10 mg can be used to prevent vomiting.

Issuing guidelines

- Negotiate the time when the pills will be taken and write it down.
- Go through the leaflet with the patient.
- Make follow-up arrangements or advise them to return to see a health professional one week after the expected date of the next period.
- Record whether emergency contraception was given or prescribed.

The insertion of a copper IUD up to five days after unprotected intercourse has an even lower failure rate (0.1%) than oral methods. It can be used up to five days after the calculated date of ovulation (i.e. the 19th day of a 28 day shortest cycle from the history, counting day 1 as the first day of bleeding) and successfully prevents implantation. The IUD can be removed at the next menstruation if it is not required or desired for continuing contraception.

Remember that exposure to unprotected intercourse means exposure to possible sexual infection also, so informed consent for screening, especially for chlamydial infection, is usually required.

LONG-ACTING CONTRACEPTION
Miss Giddy may wish to discuss her options if she wants to embark on long-acting contraception. If you have not got enough time to go through the alternatives in full detail you may supply her with leaflets or an audiotape about the possible types in Table 5.1 and arrange how she can be seen again for further advice and treatment. Don't forget to exclude pregnancy with a pregnancy test if necessary before starting her on a long-acting method. Provide the contraception at the right time of her menstrual cycle, for example,

you would give Depo-Provera, or insert an implant, within the first five days after her period has started.[10]

Female/male sterilisation

The counselling of patients is important particularly as this area is one of the commonest areas of practice leading to litigation. The RCOG has produced comprehensive evidence-based guidelines to assist practice that are essential reading for all gynaecologists.[11]

Male sterilisation

Vasectomy like female tubal occlusion is regarded as irreversible and requires a surgical procedure. It can be performed under local anaesthesia. The procedure may be carried out in a community clinic, in primary care or by urologists as opposed to gynaecologists.

Given that vasectomy does not require a general anaesthetic, it is a safer option than female tubal occlusion. It should be discussed with a woman attending for female sterilisation despite most couples having dismissed this by virtue of the fact they are seeking female sterilisation.

A no-scalpel approach is recommended because of the lower rate of early complications. Division of the vas alone has a higher failure rate than combining it with fascial interposition or diathermy, and one of these additional steps is mandatory. Clips should not be used and local anaesthesia should be used whenever possible. If there is doubt about the vas, tissue should be sent for histological confirmation.

It is advised that doctors with no previous experience should be supervised for 40 procedures (eight if they have prior surgical experience).

Operators in primary care should be able to demonstrate appropriate training and experience and have local arrangements in place with secondary care for advice or admission if required. No specific standards for facilities are required and the minimum is the same as the guidelines for minor surgery in general practice.

Post-vasectomy seminal fluid analysis is required to ensure azoospermia. It is important that the couple continue their existing form of contraception until azoospermia is confirmed. Occasionally non-motile sperm may persist some months following vasectomy. The RCOG guidelines suggest that special clearance to stop alternative contraception is acceptable if <10 000 non-motile sperm/ml are found in a fresh specimen seven months post-procedure, as no pregnancies have been reported at such a low level.[11]

Chronic testicular pain is a problem for some men following the procedure but there is no evidence of an increase in testicular cancer or cardiac disease. Reversal is possible but not always successful (and as with reversal of female sterilisation, little if any NHS funding is available). An alternative is surgical sperm recovery and intracytoplasmic sperm injections. Some men choose to freeze sperm in advance of vasectomy in case their circumstances unexpectedly change in the future.

Female sterilisation

While there is no absolute bar to offering or performing sterilisation – as long as the woman is competent to consent and there is no coercion – particular circumstances that require careful consideration include:

- young age (under 25 years)
- women without children
- sterilisation at delivery (Caesarean section)
- if there is doubt about the individual's mental capacity to consent to the procedure, in which case the decision should be referred to the courts.

Written information should be provided which the woman/couple can read at home. You should document this in the case notes.

Specific areas itemised below should be discussed.

How it is performed

Laparoscopy is the preferred approach as it is quicker and has less minor morbidity than mini-laparotomy. Mechanical occlusion by Filshie clips or rings is the method of choice. Diathermy should not be used as the primary method because of a higher risk of ectopic pregnancy and the greater difficulty in reversing it. Using more than one clip per tube routinely is not recommended. The RCOG guidelines recommend the topical application of local anaesthetic to the clips prior to application.

The risks of laparoscopy should be discussed and supported by printed leaflets that the woman (or couple) can take away and read. They should include the requirement for general anaesthetic and risk of visceral damage (approximately 1:1000) although women who are overweight or have had previous abdominal surgery are at particular risk. It should be performed as a day case wherever possible.

Discuss in advance whether the patient would accept mini-laparotomy if you encountered unexpected technical difficulties with a laparoscopic approach. (You cannot obtain this information once the patient is anaesthetised!)

The failure rate

There is a risk of 1:200 that the procedure will fail (lifetime risk), and a higher risk of ectopic pregnancy (up to 30% of pregnancies). After 10 years, the risk falls to approximately 2–3:1000. It may be useful to compare these absolute figures with vasectomy or the levonorgestrel intrauterine system (IUS).

The possibility that sterilisation is irreversible

Although sterilisation is intended to be permanent, the success of reversal should be discussed even though it is very rare for this to be funded by the NHS. Any mention of this by the patient should raise questions over the suitability of a permanent method for this couple. You should ensure that you discuss adequately alternative long-acting reversible methods of contraception.

Following the operation you should ensure that the woman knows which method was used for sterilisation. Make sure that she knows whether she needs to continue with previous contraception (e.g. continuing her oral contraception until her next period). Reiterate the importance of consulting a health professional if she thinks she may be pregnant in the future.

Sterilisation during or following pregnancy

Women should be aware of the increased regret and possible increased failure rate if the tubal occlusion is performed during or after pregnancy (whether postnatal or following termination of pregnancy). Should sterilisation be performed at the same time as Caesarean section, counselling agreement and provision of written information should have been given at least one week prior to the operation. Partial excision of the tubes (modified Pomeroy method) is recommended and histological confirmation of complete transection is advisable.

Documentation and note keeping

A preprinted checklist stamped in the patient's notes is a useful reminder in the outpatient clinic ensuring all relevant areas have been discussed including alternatives, current contraception and the importance of continuing it, at least until the procedure and possibly until the first period following sterilisation.

Trainees should perform 25 procedures under supervision before undertaking laparoscopic sterilisation independently.

Alternatives to sterilisation

Many women requesting sterilisation have poor knowledge of longer-acting methods of contraception and often opt for one of these on reflection. If either of the couple has any doubts, or if one has a life-threatening illness, one of the longer-acting methods outlined in Table 5.1 may be a more sensible choice.

Table 5.1:   Other longer-acting methods of contraception

Method	For	Against
Injection Depo-Provera (medroxyprogesterone acetate) 150 mg given intramuscularly every 12 weeks or Noristerat (norethisterone oenanthate) 200 mg every 8 weeks	• Could be started with the next period or before if pregnancy can be excluded. • Effective after seven days, possibly sooner. • Lasts for 12 weeks (or 8 weeks for Noristerat), giving time to consider longer-term action. • Usually gives very light and infrequent periods or no bleeding at all. • Enhances breast milk flow. Is likely to give very light or absent menses once breastfeeding has stopped. • Very low failure rate.	• Weight gain common with Depo-Provera, less with Noristerat. • Has to return every 12 (or 8) weeks for another injection and may easily forget unless someone else takes the responsibility for reminding her. • Progestogenic side-effects may be unacceptable: acne, feeling constantly premenstrual, irregular or absent periods. • A young woman may not have attained her peak bone mass because of her age, especially if she smokes or has a poor diet. An older woman may already have low bone mass. Depo-Provera might increase the risk of a low bone mass. • Small theoretical risk to a breast-fed baby from the absorbed progestogen, especially if a baby is premature and has immature liver enzymes.

Implant *(Implanon)*

Small plastic rod inserted in the bicipital groove of the upper arm releasing etonorgestrel over three years

- She would not require any other method for three years, giving time for reflection about her future needs.
- If someone in the practice fits implants, she could have one fitted within 5 days of the start of her next period.
- She does not have to remember anything for three years.
  Very low failure rate.

- Usually cannot be done immediately and needs some time to set up a fitting.
- If no one in practice fits these, patient may have to attend another venue.
- Frequent spotting or light periods may not suit everyone and a few people have unacceptable progestogenic side-effects.
- Recall system needed so that the implant is not forgotten.

Intrauterine device with copper *(IUCD)*

Cu T380 Multiload 350
Nova-T380 Flexi-T

- Could be fitted immediately if facilities available and pregnancy can be excluded.
- Would give protection between 5–10 years depending on device.
- Cu T380 has a very low failure rate with the others only slightly higher.
- Can be used as a post-coital method if she is at risk following unprotected intercourse.

- Might have to re-attend or attend a different venue if no facilities to fit it immediately.
- Easier to fit in the multiparous uterus.
- Success rates dependent more on the expertise of the person fitting it than on the type of device used. Health professionals who only fit a few devices each year have higher expulsion, bleeding, removal and perforation rates.
- Usually increases the menstrual loss and may increase dysmenorrhoea if present.
- Recall system needed so that it is not forgotten.

Intrauterine system with progesterone *(IUS)*

Mirena

- Could be fitted within 5 days of the start of her next period if facilities are available.
- Decreases menstrual loss, usually to none after first few months of irregular loss.

- Might have to re-attend or attend a different venue if no facilities to fit it immediately.
- Nulliparous women usually need cervical anaesthesia as the diameter of the device is wider than an IUD.

Table 5.1:   Continued

Method	For	Against
	• Would give protection for 5 years. • Failure rate is even lower than sterilisation.	• Success rates dependent more on the expertise of the person fitting it than on the type of device used. Specific training needed as different insertion technique to other IUCDs. • Decreases menstrual loss, usually to none after first few months of irregular loss. • Recall system needed so that it is not forgotten.
Combined contraceptive patch	• Only needs application weekly for three weeks, omitted for the fourth week. • Good cycle control. • Under the control of the woman if she wants to stop it at any time. • Low failure rate but not as low as any of the methods above.	• The oestrogen component can reduce breast milk flow. • The oestrogen component increases her thrombosis risk. • She has to remember it weekly. • It is expensive compared with oral contraceptive pill.

Case study 5.2

Mrs Fecund is aged 32, and 14 weeks pregnant in her third pregnancy. Her two previous pregnancies have resulted in live births. Her children are aged 8 and 4 respectively. Both deliveries were by Caesarean section and an elective Caesarean section is planned for 39 weeks' gestation – she is requesting sterilisation.

What issues you should cover

As the mode of delivery has been decided at booking, the main issue is whether to agree to sterilisation at this procedure given the higher failure rate with sterilisation in pregnancy. The option of sterilisation some months following delivery should be discussed. Discussing loss of an existing child or of the current pregnancy can be upsetting but as mortality is highest in the first year of life this will concentrate the couple's mind on whether it really is the best time to be sterilised.

If sterilisation is undertaken, it is recommended that a modified Pomeroy method is used (physically excising a portion of each tube), as this has a lower failure rate than the application of Filshie clips. The excised fallopian tube should be sent for histology to confirm complete transection.

Discuss sterilisation at least one week prior to delivery and provide written information. Clear documentation within the case records is essential. There is no guidance on what should be recommended if she requires preterm delivery but in circumstances where the neonatal outlook is uncertain, *not* proceeding with sterilisation appears advisable.

Termination of pregnancy

Termination of pregnancy is a common request. There is a legal requirement that two medical practitioners agree to the termination of pregnancy and that they both sign a form (Schedule A) with the indication for termination as outlined in The Abortion Act of 1967.[12] A minority of terminations are carried out for severe maternal medical conditions that involve risk to the woman's life in continuing the pregnancy (e.g. severe cardiac disease) or for fetal abnormality (chromosomal or structural abnormality on ultrasound). Most terminations are carried out under criterion 3:

> The continuance of the pregnancy would involve risk, greater than if the pregnancy were terminated, of injury to the physical or mental health of the pregnant woman.

As termination of pregnancy is safer than continuing to term and delivering, this clause can be invoked to cater for most women who ask for a termination.

Some doctors working in reproductive medicine may not wish to be involved in terminations on ethical or religious grounds and this is accepted and respected. Doctors who have opted out of termination care should refer on to other practitioners promptly if they are asked for their clinical opinion.

It is essential that the woman is adequately counselled about her options and receives information on the benefits and risks associated with each method. It is important to be non-directional and provide reliable information to enable the woman to reach her own decision. Take blood for grouping and endocervical swabs. Treat infection before the termination is carried out and remember contact tracing. You may need to give anti-D. Consult the guidelines about what actions you should take.[13] Follow-up and future contraceptive plans should be arranged.

Methods include medical or surgical termination of pregnancy. The use of mifepristone (anti-progesterone) combined with prostaglandin analogues (up to 63 days amenorrhea) in the first trimester provides an effective alternative to surgical evacuation of the uterus under general anaesthesia. Surgical terminations are done under local anaesthesia in some centres. Medical termination is usually performed up to 12 weeks with pre-operative cervical preparation of cervix (prostaglandin analogues Misoprostol or Dinoprost) aiding dilation. Second trimester terminations at more advanced gestations are usually performed medically although practitioners experienced in dilatation and evacuation have undertaken surgical evacuations at gestations of up to 16–18 weeks.

Complications following termination include retained products of conception (up to 5%) requiring further surgery. As the retained products may be infected, give antibiotics for 24 h before surgery. Adequate treatment of existing, often asymptomatic, infection (detected by cervical and vaginal swabs) should reduce the risk of pelvic inflammatory disease following termination. Surgical evacuation carries a small risk of uterine perforation. Longer-term consequences such as regret and guilt over the decision are uncommon and may be minimised by adequate counselling pre-termination.[14]

Women who present with subfertility following a pregnancy (including termination) should have early investigation of tubal patency because of possible damage by infection.

Contraception and termination in under-16 year olds

Teenage women who become pregnant have a higher maternal and perinatal mortality. This is particularly marked in the under-16s and is associated with poor education, cigarette smoking, poor nutrition and deprivation.

Women younger than 16 years can have emergency contraception or a termination of pregnancy without parental consent but take great care to ensure that she is competent to give consent (*see* Box 5.1).

Collecting data to demonstrate your learning, competence, performance and standards of service delivery

Example cycle of evidence 5.1

- Focus: clinical care
- Other relevant focus: probity

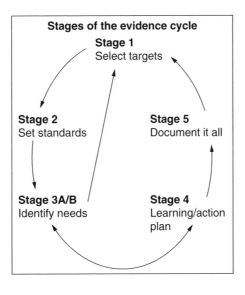

Case study 5.3

Miss Chance is a 15 year old who attends on a Friday evening to see the practice nurse on duty. The girl's mother is one of the morning receptionists at the surgery. This is the second week since starting work at the practice three months ago that this nurse has been working on her own in the treatment suite. The nurse is aware that you have a special interest in reproductive health, so she contacts you to ask if she can give her some emergency contraceptive pills from the stock in the treatment room. The nurse has not done any family planning training but tells you she thinks she can go through the protocol she has been told is on the computer, if you would like her to try.

You have not previously assessed the competency of the practice nurse to do this task. It is not safe to assume that she will perform adequately, nor is it fair to give her this responsibility without training. She may be offering to do something outside her limits of competency because 'she does not know what she does not know'. She may also be pressurised by the patient for a quick solution because of the relationship with one of the receptionists. The patient should not receive inferior care just because she is the daughter of a member of staff.

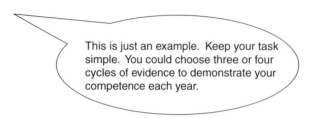

This is just an example. Keep your task simple. You could choose three or four cycles of evidence to demonstrate your competence each year.

Stage 1: Select your aspirations for good practice

The excellent doctor:

- responds rapidly to emergencies
- arranges appropriate training for staff in managing emergencies.

Stage 2: Set the standards for your outcomes

Outcomes might include:

- the way learning is applied
- a learnt skill
- a protocol
- a strategy that is implemented
- meeting recommended standards.

- Demonstrate consistent best practice in provision of emergency contraception to teenagers in respect of availability and accessibility and clinical management.
- Demonstrate best practice in the maintenance of confidentiality.
- Information about contraceptive services you provide, e.g. in the practice leaflet, is factual and verifiable, conforms with the law and with guidance issued by the Advertising Standards Authority.
- Information that you publish about the quality of your contraceptive services can be justified (e.g. that you do not claim that IUDs or vasectomies can be done at any time if patients have to make specific arrangements for that service).

- Information published about your services does not exploit patients' vulnerability or lack of medical knowledge or put pressure on people to use a service.

Stage 3A: Identify your learning needs

- Carry out with other staff a significant event audit e.g. a teenager who became pregnant after consulting you about contraception three months previously. This may throw up learning needs about emergency contraception (*see* Box 5.2) or about actively listening to patients.
- Record in your own reflective diary trends or comments relating to problems or issues of emergency contraception in teenagers. This might be to do with how well the services are running or about consultations with you or other doctors or nurses.
- Do a notes review to audit how often you discuss, and screen for, STIs. Exposure to unprotected intercourse is exposure to infection (unless within a monogamous partnership).
- Audit your own adherence to the protocol for emergency contraception.

Stage 3B: Identify your service needs

Any of the needs assessment exercises in 3A may also reveal service needs.

- Audit the accessibility of aspects of family planning services e.g. a patient survey to establish the interval between the time an appointment is requested by a teenager to making face-to-face contact with a nurse or doctor. You may establish that this new practice nurse requires training in family planning to supplement the availability of present staff, or that there are sufficient trained staff to cope with most of the demand.
- Observe the pathway of care received e.g. by a pregnant teenager who had presented to the reception at her GP's surgery or community clinic either before, or more than, 72 h after unprotected sex.
- Check with staff that everyone is aware of the need for confidentiality, and how it should be maintained, e.g. the manager might use this case (anonymously) to illustrate the pitfalls, and that no one should inadvertently mention seeing someone at the surgery or clinic.
- Ask the PCO or other external commentators to critique the information you supply about your contraceptive services (practice or clinic leaflet or other published information).

Stage 4: Make and carry out a learning and action plan

- Read up on latest recommendations for emergency contraception and revise the protocol if required.
- Read up and discuss at a practice meeting the latest evidence about progestogen-only emergency contraception. You might want to be an innovator and extend the time limits for giving it from 72 h to five days.[15]
- Visit other services where there is excellent practice in delivering appropriate care for teenagers and/or contraceptive services.

Stage 5: Document your learning, competence, performance and standards of service delivery

- Re-audit the consistent application of policy or protocol relating to emergency contraception.
- Repeat the teenage patient survey for timely access.
- Repeat your reflective diary.
- Audit the awareness of staff with a checklist about confidentiality.
- Include the practice or clinic leaflet describing services provided.

Case study 5.3 continued

You see Miss Chance yourself, and assess her need for emergency contraception. You should ensure that her confidentiality is assured. She is only just within the 72-hour limit for emergency contraception but does not want to have an IUD fitted. You give her both the Levonelle-2 pills immediately from your emergency stock. You discuss using continuing contraception, but she says she does not need it. You ask her to return to see you if she changes her mind and reassure her again about confidentiality. You discuss ways she might talk about her future needs for continuing contraception at home. You also give her a leaflet about the opening times and contact telephone numbers of the local clinics in case she would prefer to attend there. You remind the staff on duty about confidentiality.

Example cycle of evidence 5.2

- Focus: clinical care
- Other relevant focus: teaching and training

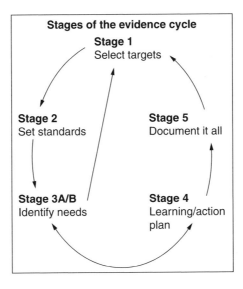

Stages of the evidence cycle

Stage 1
Select targets

Stage 2
Set standards

Stage 5
Document it all

Stage 3A/B
Identify needs

Stage 4
Learning/action
plan

Case study 5.4

Mrs Daffy tells the SHO working in your gynaecology clinic that her husband says she must be sterilised. She delivered her fifth child six weeks ago and has had two miscarriages as well. She has been prescribed some progestogen-only pills to start on the 21st day after delivery but says she has not had time to obtain them from the pharmacy yet. She adds that she doesn't like taking pills anyway. She is obviously overweight and from her medical record it can be seen that she is 29 years old, smokes but has a normal blood pressure. She asks if it is okay to breastfeed the baby who is crying loudly, and two of her other children start investigating the drawers and cupboards in the consulting room. This is the first clinic session that the SHO has taken and he turns to you looking completely overwhelmed.

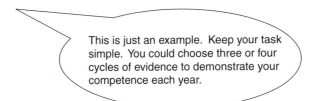

This is just an example. Keep your task simple. You could choose three or four cycles of evidence to demonstrate your competence each year.

Stage 1: Select your aspirations for good practice

The excellent doctor:

- makes an adequate assessment of the patient's condition, based on the history and, if indicated, an appropriate examination
- provides or arranges investigations or treatment where necessary
- recognises and works within the limits of his/her competence and refers to another practitioner when indicated
- consults with colleagues and keeps them informed when sharing the care of patients.

Stage 2: Set the standards for your outcomes

Outcomes might include:

- the way learning is applied
- a learnt skill
- a protocol
- a strategy that is implemented
- meeting recommended standards.

- Demonstrate consistent best practice in provision of continuing contraception to patients in respect of availability and accessibility and clinical management.
- Demonstrate best use of resources.
- Contribute to the education of students or colleagues willingly.
- Develop the skills, attitudes and practices of a competent teacher if you have responsibilities for teaching.
- Ensure that students and junior colleagues are properly supervised in line with the responsibilities you have for teaching them.

Stage 3A: Identify your learning needs

- Carry out a significant event audit with other staff e.g. looking at the reasons why Mrs Daffy or a similar patient had not used contraception previously. Had she defaulted from care or had there been failures in the system or standards of care?
- Examine a complaint e.g. about inadequate counselling before sterilisation or vasectomy. Do you need to use an up-to-date leaflet or a checklist to ensure that people have sufficient information to make an informed choice?

- Keep a reflective diary capturing trends or comments relating to problems or issues of longer-acting methods of contraception e.g. you might record that you no longer feel competent doing IUD or IUS fittings because of changes in devices and lack of practice due to low demand. You may want to provide implant fittings but lack the training.
- Ask for feedback from the SHO about the effectiveness of the supervision and whether he felt supported sufficiently during his steep learning curve in the realities of dealing with demanding patients in a gynaecology clinic.

Stage 3B: Identify your service needs

Any of the needs assessment exercises in 3A may also reveal service needs.

- Review the difficulty of finding the time to fit an IUD or IUS because of competing demands on your own time, or the limited availability of local family planning services.
- Perform a patient survey to ascertain the demand and when people would like to be able to access a service providing longer-acting methods.
- Audit the availability and adequacy of emergency resuscitation equipment and the training standards of health professionals to use it.
- Identify the SHO's learning style and what learning tasks you set to match his style.

Stage 4: Make and carry out a learning and action plan

- Consider a refresher course and practical training on modern IUD and IUS fitting. Learn how to fit and remove implants.
- Research the availability of provision of longer-acting methods of contraception and liaise with those services. Perhaps you might help to make a proposal to the PCO for more accessible local provision. This might involve finding out the comparative costs of various contraceptive options.
- Read up about alternative methods of contraception and the points to consider about sterilisation counselling.

Stage 5: Document your learning, competence, performance and standards of service delivery

- Retain any certificates of learning and competence achieved.
- Record and disseminate your learning about other contraceptive provision.
- Record a log of IUD and IUS fittings and their outcomes.

- Record changes you have made to your provision of contraception in your reflective diary.
- Re-audit the availability and adequacy of emergency resuscitation equipment after any necessary changes have been made, and also record the training standards of health professionals who use it.
- Record that you set aside a longer appointment time for patients (with their consent) because you were teaching e.g. demonstrating counselling and insertion techniques for an IUD or implant fitting as in the case study.
- Record how you helped the SHO learn from managing Mrs Daffy himself, rather than just taking over completely yourself.

Case study 5.4 continued

It is clearly impossible to undertake an adequate medical assessment initially. Help the SHO to arrange with Mrs Daffy for someone to look after the children while he does this assessment. If it is beyond the limits of the SHO's competence, he may need to refer Mrs Daffy to another health professional for contraceptive treatment.

Mrs Daffy refuses the offer of an immediate injection or pill. She is able to get her sister to look after the older children, while she just brings the baby to the clinic. One of the receptionists is able to look after the baby after he has been fed and is in his pushchair. The SHO is able to have a full discussion of the options for contraception. She says her husband would never 'be done'. She decides she definitely wants an IUS after all the advantages and disadvantages are explained. She is keen for the SHO to see the IUS fitting which is arranged in the family planning clinic the following week.

The SHO will probably want to discuss Mrs Daffy's situation with the health visitor and should ask her for permission to do so. Other professionals, such as a social worker, might be involved with the family.

Example cycle of evidence 5.3

- Focus: maintaining good medical practice

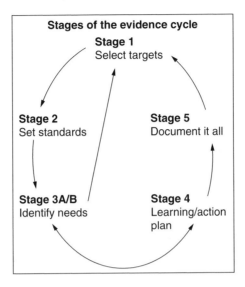

Stages of the evidence cycle

Stage 1
Select targets

Stage 2
Set standards

Stage 5
Document it all

Stage 3A/B
Identify needs

Stage 4
Learning/action
plan

Case study 5.5

A slim 37-year-old non-smoker is referred to the gynaecological clinic with anaemia secondary to heavy regular menses. She is in a new relationship and mentions she is not happy with her boyfriend using barrier methods for contraception. Sometimes he forgets to use a condom and she is very frightened that she might become pregnant.

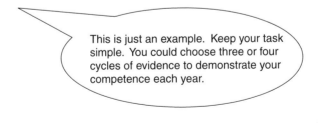

This is just an example. Keep your task simple. You could choose three or four cycles of evidence to demonstrate your competence each year.

Stage 1: Select your aspirations for good practice

The excellent doctor:

- considers both the gynaecological problem and her dissatisfaction with her current contraception
- excludes serious underlying pathology before considering treatment
- discusses all management options that may improve menstrual loss and provide contraception (e.g. surgical, hormonal contraception and the Mirena IUS)
- develops a management plan in consultation with the patient, considering individual priorities and circumstances.

Stage 2: Set the standards for your outcomes

Outcomes might include:

- the way learning is applied
- a learnt skill
- a protocol
- a strategy that is implemented
- meeting recommended standards.

- Demonstrate best practice in the assessment and management of menorrhagia.
- Demonstrate understanding of contraceptive choices.

Stage 3A: Identify your learning needs

- Do you have sufficient knowledge of the effectiveness, benefits, drawbacks and cautions of various contraceptive options so that you may advise patients appropriately?
- Do you have a systematic approach to the management of menorrhagia?
- Review the management of your last 10 patients with menorrhagia, considering their contraceptive needs and how these were met.

Stage 3B: Identify your service needs

Any of the needs assessment exercises in 3A may also reveal service needs.

- Review the use of transvaginal ultrasound and endometrial sampling for women referred with menorrhagia.
- Audit the number of outpatient visits to your gynaecology clinic for each patient with menorrhagia and consider whether the number of visits may be reduced.
- Survey patients' views on the advice they have received about menorrhagia and enquire how this may be improved.

Stage 4: Make and carry out a learning and action plan

- Reflect on your understanding of the modern management of menorrhagia. Attend a relevant lecture or full meeting and review the RCOG guidelines[16] and read up on both medical and surgical management options.
- Discuss local contraceptive options with the lead of a local family planning centre. Perhaps consider attendance at several family planning clinics to refresh your contraceptive knowledge and optimal patient counselling about contraception.
- Consider setting up a one-stop clinic with access to transvaginal ultrasound, hysteroscopy and endometrial sampling and levonorgestrel-containing IUS.

Stage 5: Document your learning, competence, performance and standards of service delivery

- File your notes summarising your update on menorrhagia management with any attendance certificates for any relevant lectures. Present what you have learnt to your colleagues and keep a record of this presentation.
- Keep a record of the last 10 patients you managed with menorrhagia and the eventual outcome.
- Produce a series of local guidelines to help advise on the management of menorrhagia, including contraceptive guidance and patient information leaflets.

Case study 5.5 continued

Transvaginal ultrasonography and endometrial sampling reveal no abnormalities suggesting the patient has dysfunctional menstrual bleeding. Although the patient does not wish to become pregnant at this early stage in her new relationship, she considers that she may wish to have a child later. She is thus relieved to discover her menses could be improved without compromising her possibility of later pregnancy. Following discussion of possible options to reduce menstrual blood loss and provide reliable contraception the patient chooses to have a Mirena coil.

References

1   The Fraser Guidelines (1985) House of Lords Judgement, London. www.dh.gov.uk/assetRoot/04/08/69/14/04086914.pdf

2   Department of Health (1999) *Teenage Pregnancy*. Social Exclusion Unit, Department of Health, London.

3   Chambers R, Wakley G and Chambers S (2001) *Tackling Teenage Pregnancy: sex culture and needs*. Radcliffe Medical Press, Oxford.

4   Acheson D (chair) (1998) *Independent Inquiry into Inequalities in Health Report*. The Stationery Office, London.

5   The general leaflet *Contraception*, those on individual methods, and a good range of other leaflets, are available from fpa, 2–12 Pentonville Road, London N1 9FP, UK. Tel: +44 (0)20 7837 5432.

6   World Health Organization (2000) *Improving Access to Quality Care in Family Planning*. WHO, Geneva. www.who.int/reproductive-health

7   Website for the Faculty of Family Planning and Reproductive Health Care. www.ffprhc.org.uk/

8   Faculty of Family Planning and Reproductive Health Care: Clinical Effectiveness Unit (2003) FFPRHC Guidance: Emergency contraception. *Journal of Family Planning and Reproductive Health Care*. **29**: 9–16. www.ffprhc.org.uk (publications).

9   Trussel J (1998) Contraceptive efficacy. In: J Trussel, F Stewart, W Cates *et al.* (eds) *Contraceptive Technology* (17e). Ardent Media, New York.

10 Belfield T (1999) *Contraceptive Handbook* (3e). Family Planning Association, London.

11 Royal College of Obstetricians and Gynaecologists (2004) *Male and Female Sterilisation*. RCOG Press, London. www.rcog.org.uk/resources/Public/Sterilisation_full.pdf

12 Abortion Legislation. http://www.btinternet.com/~DEvans_23/legislat.htm

13 National electronic Library for Health. *The Care of Women Requesting Induced Abortion*. www.nelh.nhs.uk/guidelinesdb/html/fulltext-introduction/Induced Abortion.html

14 Hodson P and Seber P (2002) A woman's right to choose … counselling! *Journal of Family Planning and Reproductive Health Care*. **28**: 174–5.

15 Ellertson C, Evans M, Ferden S *et al.* (2003) Extending the time limit for starting the Yupze regimen of emergency contraception to 120 hours. *Obstetrics and Gynecology*. **101**: 1168–71.

16 Royal College of Obstetricians and Gynaecologists (RCOG) Guidelines on the initial management of menorrhagia. http://www.rcog.org.uk/guidelines.asp?pageID=108&GuidelineID=28

Further reading

- Belfield T (1999) *Contraceptive Handbook* (3e). Family Planning Association, London.
- Glasier A and Gebbie A (2000) *Handbook of Family Planning and Reproductive Health Care.* Churchill Livingstone, London.
- Guillebaud J (2003) *Contraception: your questions answered* (4e). Churchill Livingstone, London.
- Royal College of Obstetricians and Gynaecologists (2004) *Male and Female Sterilisation.* Royal College of Obstetricians and Gynaecologists, London.
- Trussell J, Stewart F, Cates W *et al.* (1998) *Contraceptive Technology* (17e). Ardent Media, New York.
- Wakley G and Chambers R (2002) *Sexual Health Matters in Primary Care.* Radcliffe Medical Press, Oxford.
- Wakley G, Cunnion M and Chambers R (2003) *Improving Sexual Health Advice in Primary Care and Beyond.* Radcliffe Medical Press, Oxford.

6

Sexually transmitted infections

Although specialist care for STIs is provided in genitourinary medicine (GUM) clinics, patients may present with STIs in primary care, in hospital accident and emergency departments, as acute gynaecological emergencies and to gynaecology clinics. Anyone practising in the field of reproductive health needs a grounding in STIs. This chapter will start with presentation in primary care and move onto the scenario of an acute hospital admission.

Case study 6.1

A 21-year-old woman attends telling you that her recent ex-partner has sent her a text message accusing her of giving him an infection. She has little other information except that he has been to the GUM clinic in the next town. She refuses to attend the GUM clinic and wants you to treat her as she has heard that you have special interest in reproductive health.

What issues you should cover[1]

Giving information about GUM clinics

Access to GUM clinics varies across the country and new users often find it difficult to know what is available. People are often fearful of attending because of perceived stigma, or just because going somewhere new always provokes anxiety – and it is difficult to ask a friend to go with them for support. You should know where the clinics are and how people can be seen. Some clinics have open access while others require appointments to be made by telephone. Some are open in the evening, others from 10 am to 5 pm (not very convenient!). Some of the clinics now have a seamless one-stop service together with contraceptive clinics or are on the same premises to allow for easy transfers between services.

Stress that the service is confidential and that the records are kept separately from other hospital records. By law, staff in a GUM clinic cannot tell a patient if or what STI their partner has, or tell their doctor that they have attended unless the patient requests it. The clinic cannot give any information to other doctors, solicitors, insurance companies or the police without the consent of the patient. The clinic will record a name and a date of birth, and will ask for a contact address so that results can be given (but patients do not have to give this information if they prefer not to).

After a detailed history, often using a checklist, tests can be done immediately to diagnose some infections. Other tests will take some time for the results to be known. The clinic does need some identifying information so that they can access patients' records when they re-attend. All treatment is free of charge and this can be a potent incentive to attend if treatment is needed. Reimbursement of travel expenses can also sometimes be made.

The patient needs to be clear that you will not be able to give such a complete service away from the GUM clinic, partly because of the limitations for carrying out testing. Results of testing are more reliable if the patient travels to the hospital laboratory with her samples still in her in the body than if you take samples and transport them separately. The pick up rate from samples falls the longer the delay between testing and examination of the specimens.

Taking a sexual history[1]

If she still refuses to attend the GUM clinic, then you must do your best for her. Explain the reason for taking a sexual history. This reduces the possibility that the patient will be offended or misinterpret your intentions. Ask the patient if it is all right to carry on.

Tell the patient about confidentiality – mention this early on and explain how the information given will be kept confidential and who will have access to that information. Consider asking their partner to participate or to supply information if the patient agrees (unlikely in this case). If a partner does attend, allow for one-to-one discussion, as some issues involve sexual activity with other partners or information that one of a couple would not want the other to hear.

Listen carefully – allow the patient to guide the discussion and introduce the terminology. This does not imply that you should use the same language or slang as patients do. Be careful about the words that you and the patient use. The vagina or uterus mean something specific to you, but the terms may be used in a much wider sense by patients to indicate any part of the female genitals. Similarly, someone may talk about 'going to bed with someone' and you need to be clear whether this actually includes sexual penetration. 'Making love' may include sexual penetration, or may refer to caressing and other sexual stimulation. There are problems too with identifying the sex of the partner, 'Pat' or 'Lesley' could be either. Always check that what you understand is what the patient meant.

Ask the patient to tell you about her sexual activity. Give examples e.g. 'have you had oral sex?' Explain each time why you are asking those questions. Other forms of sexual activity should also be specified, depending on the patient's sexual orientation. You will need to know the areas of the body that might become infected (throat, rectum, etc) so that investigations are complete but relevant.

Ask about symptoms, but bear in mind (and tell the patient) that most people with an STI do not have any symptoms. Has she had any burning when she passes water, any change in her vaginal secretions, any soreness, rash or lumps in the genital area or any irregular bleeding between the periods or after intercourse? Has there been any change in the amount of her period loss or any episodes of abdominal pain?

Enquire about any previous STI and her own perception of her risk. An estimate can be made from the length of time she was with that partner and how many other sexual partners she has had in the last 12 months.

Giving information about STIs

You need to find out what she knows about STIs. She may be reluctant to have any investigations performed if she has no symptoms. You can give her some information about how often people are infected in her age group and about her risks – adjusted for her level of comprehension. Then she will be in a better position to make an informed choice.

Statistics about STIs[2]

- Cases of chlamydia trachomatis identified have doubled in the last six years. In 2002, genital chlamydial infection was the commonest bacterial STI seen. Highest rates of diagnosis of chlamydia are seen in young people, particularly women in the 16 to 19 year and 20 to 24 year age groups.
- Genital warts (HPV) are the commonest viral STI and also the commonest STI overall.
- Gonorrhoea (GC): the rise in the number of cases of gonorrhoea has been largest in the youngest age groups – 16 to 19 years and 20 to 24 years of age. The majority of cases identified have been in men – largely because women rarely have symptoms. The recent slight fall in rates recently is thought to be due to better treatment of strains resistant to commonly used antibiotics.
- HIV infection rates continue to rise. HIV infection is now identified more commonly in heterosexuals than in homosexual men. Infection rates are increasing, perhaps due to a relaxation of the vigilance of people who

believed that they were at risk and used condoms after publicity campaigns, but have now become complacent about the risk, as it is no longer in the news.

- Hepatitis B rates have slightly decreased but hepatitis C rates have increased, perhaps reflecting the effect of immunisation against hepatitis B.
- Some other infections that occur elsewhere in the body such as streptococcus (that usually causes skin and throat infections), or gut bacteria like *E. coli*, can be spread by sexual activity. Molluscum contagiosum is a very common infection, especially in children but can also be spread through sexual activity. Some other more unusual STIs may be seen occasionally in people returning from other countries.
- Although thrush and bacterial vaginosis are not classified as STIs, they are common causes of genital infection. Thrush (also known as candida, or candidiasis) is not usually passed on from a woman to a man by sexual intercourse. It is a very common cause of vaginal discharge, soreness and itching. Bacterial vaginosis is possibly even more frequently found in women complaining of vaginal discharge.

Knowledge about the individual infections[3]

Ask her what she knows about the infections to find out what other information she might need.

Chlamydia

In under-26 year olds, chlamydia has been identified in about 10–12% of people in studies of population screening. Chlamydial infection is frequently asymptomatic but is a common cause of infertility and chronic pelvic infection. It can cause ectopic pregnancy and chronic pelvic pain. Ascending infection in men causes epididymitis but evidence of male infertility is limited. Maternal to infant transmission causes neonatal conjunctivitis and pneumonia. It may co-exist with other STIs and may help in the transmission and acquisition of HIV infection.

Gonorrhoea

The incidence of this infection has been increasing especially among 16–19 year olds. Infection can be asymptomatic in about 10% of men and 50% of women. Male symptoms of dysuria, discharge or epididymitis, or female symptoms of discharge, dysuria or abdominal pain should raise your suspicions.

Non-specific urethritis or non-specific genital infection

This is common in young men and is defined as an infection, usually urethritis, not caused by gonorrhoea. Up to 40% of episodes of urethritis are in fact caused by chlamydia, so she will need tests for this. *Mycoplasma genitalium* and

Ureaplasma urealyticum are commonest amongst the other causative organisms. The diagnosis is mainly made by a combination of symptoms of urethritis and the presence of pus cells – more than five per high power field (×400) – on a slide made from a urethral swab. The male partner will have been told to get his partner(s) treated to prevent recurrence. Treatment is as for chlamydia.

Genital warts – human papilloma virus (HPV)

First ever presentation of genital warts has shown a significant rise in the 16–19-year-old age group. HPV infection is common amongst sexually active young people whether or not visible warts are present. Small plane warts may be visible on examination without any symptoms being present. Genital warts are usually spread sexually, so their presence should prompt a search for other STIs. Some HPVs (types 16, 18, 31, 33 and 35) – not usually the ones presenting as visible warts – are associated with the development of cervical cancer and yearly cervical screening for five years is normally suggested if wart virus is found. Determining the type of HPV present is still a research technique.

Syphilis

Although many people know that syphilis is an STI, new cases of syphilis in the UK are uncommon and are mostly found by screening in pregnancy or on blood donation. The presence of a solitary ulcer or the rash of secondary syphilis may raise suspicions.

Viral hepatitis

Several different virus types cause hepatitis, all of which can cause an acute illness with jaundice. Asymptomatic infections are common. Hepatitis B and D also cause chronic infection progressing to cirrhosis and liver failure. Hepatitis B is more infectious than human immunodeficiency virus (HIV) and can be spread by sexual intercourse as well as from contaminated blood. Hepatitis A can be caught sexually from a partner with an active infection.

Human immunodeficiency disease (HIV)

The symptoms of an acute infection with HIV may resemble glandular fever, but most new infections do not show any symptoms. The development of antibodies after infection takes about two to six weeks, but can be later than this. Chronic infection may also be asymptomatic, but about one-third of patients have generalised persistently enlarged lymph nodes. Later in the course of the chronic infection symptoms of night sweats, fevers, diarrhoea and weight loss occur. Frequent infections of mucous membranes or skin are often present. About 75% of HIV-positive individuals develop symptoms over a 9–10 year period without therapy.

Trichomonas vaginalis

This organism with a flagella occurs in the urethra in both genders but also in the vagina and paraurethral glands in women. In adults it is a STI and is frequently associated with other STIs. (Babies can acquire the infection perinatally from an infected mother.) The commonest complaint in both men and women is of discharge, but 15–50% of men have no symptoms. Women also complain of itching, dysuria or a smelly discharge. Although the discharge is classically described as frothy yellow, it is often variable both in consistency and colour.

Bacterial vaginosis (BV)

BV may be even more common than 'thrush'. It was formerly called 'Gardnerella vaginosis' and is the overgrowth of predominately anaerobic bacteria that are normally present in only small numbers in the healthy vagina. They produce a fishy or ammonia smell in alkaline conditions so the condition may be worse after intercourse or just after a woman's periods have finished.

BV is causing increasing concern to health professionals because of:

- pelvic inflammatory disease
- endometritis
- post-operative cuff infection after a transabdominal hysterectomy (TAH) and vaginal hysterectomy
- post-abortal infection
- psychosexual problems (the smell!)
- obstetric factors: increase in late miscarriage rates, chorioendometritis, preterm delivery
- as a possible co-factor in HIV transmission.

Thrush

Sometimes this fungal infection may be reported on cervical smears or swabs taken for other reasons when there are no symptoms. The first attack can be extremely uncomfortable with the swelling, itching, soreness and discharge causing considerable distress. Although often described as typically presenting with white 'cottage cheese'-like patches over bright red areas of the vulval or vaginal walls, this is more frequent in pregnancy. The appearance of the discharge may be very variable and the vulva may be fissured or red and shiny from frequent scratching. Most women complain mainly of:

- itching and soreness
- rapid onset often in the premenstrual week
- painful urination and/or sexual intercourse.

Investigations that may be needed

You need to discuss with the woman what tests you can do, how long the results will take and how she will obtain the results. She may be happy for you to contact her at home but, if not, other arrangements must be made such as sending them to a trusted friend. If she does not give consent to be contacted then it is essential that she understands that she must re-attend for the results. Investigations that could be carried out are shown in Table 6.1.

Table 6.1: Suggested investigations for screening for an STI indicated by the history

Test	Useful for
HVS in Stuart's or similar transport medium	candida, bacterial vaginosis, trichomonas
Cervical exudate swab or endocervical swab and urethral swab in Stuart's or similar transport medium	gram stain shows gram negative diplococcus in about half of all gonococcal infections; culture as well will detect about 90% of infections
Chlamydia test Know which testing procedure your microbiology department uses. If it is enzyme immunoassay (EIA) send an endocervical swab and urethral swab. Use the special chlamydial testing kit supplied by your laboratory for taking samples from the cervix. Follow the instructions that come with the pack from the laboratory as each type of pack has different instructions. Some are very clear and state that the cleaning swab (the large bulbous swab of the two) must not be used as the swab for chlamydia. First clean any mucus off the cervix with the cleaning swab and then use the chlamydia swab (the metal or plastic handled, thin flat ended swab). Rotate it for a minimum of 30 seconds in the cervix. Take cells from the transitional zone (the junction between the outer cells of the cervix and the inner ones lining the cervical canal). Remove the swab from the vagina and place it in the container supplied in accordance with the instructions	chlamydia trachomatis
First catch urine (not MSU)	nucleic acid amplification tests for chlamydia trachomatis and/or gonorrhoea*
Viral swabs from any ulcers or sores	herpes simplex, candida
Swabs from other sites e.g. pharynx, rectum	gonococcus
Blood test	viral hepatitis or HIV

*Nucleic acid amplification tests have been developed that are highly sensitive (over 90%) compared with the standard endocervical enzyme immunoassay (EIA) test that has a lower sensitivity of 60–70%. You will need to know what the standards are for your laboratory and their specificity rate (so that you know how many false-positive and false-negative results might be expected).

Prevention of transmission[4]

It is important to ensure that any infection is not spread to any other partner(s). Partner notification is an important part of the control of STIs but is often difficult to achieve. The woman should be advised to abstain from intercourse until she has been screened and treated. Remember not all women are able to refuse to have sexual intercourse if there is an imbalance of power between the partners, or if cultural or religious customs prevent her expressing her wishes.

Treatment[5]

If you can establish what infection her previous partner has been told he has, treatment for this infection could be started as soon as investigations are complete. She should only be treated empirically if you cannot obtain her consent to investigations. It is possible for her to have an infection that has not been identified in her previous partner. The reasons for this can be either he has not contracted an infection that she has, or because of the limitations of the test (that is, he has had a false-negative test).

General principles to consider when introducing screening of well people for illnesses or infections

Case study 6.1 continued

Before she leaves the patient asks you why she was not screened for infections like chlamydia when she had her recent cervical smear. You tell her a little of what is described in Box 6.1 and the general principles of screening with special regard to chlamydia.

Box 6.1:   General principles to consider when screening for illnesses or infections

- *Is the condition important?* Chlamydia is an important cause of infertility, ectopic pregnancy, salpingitis, chronic pelvic pain and morbidity.
- *Is the natural history well understood?* Between 70 and 80% of women have cervical infections with no symptoms, but it is not clear how many have a risk of ascending infections in the absence of precipitating factors such as instrumentation of the uterus.
- *Is there a recognisable early stage?* Screening tests can identify infection when no symptoms are present.
- *Is there a suitable test?* The nucleic acid amplification tests are more sensitive and specific than the previous EIA tests and can be done on urine as well as swabs. Blood tests are not useful as they tell you only if someone has ever had the infection (and possibly got rid of it), not whether they have it currently.
- *Is the test acceptable?* Urine tests are more acceptable than cervical or urethral swabs. Self-taken swabs have also been shown to be useful and acceptable in some groups.
- *At what intervals should the test be repeated?* This is unknown – and may depend on the accuracy and completeness of contact tracing and treatment, and on social factors like change of sexual partner or monogamy.
- *Are there adequate facilities for the diagnosis and treatment?* No: primary care health professionals do not always have sufficient time or skills or facilities for investigation, GUM clinics need increased resources to cope with the number of referrals of people with positive tests and the laboratories have insufficient capacity and resources to carry out the tests. Instigating a campaign about chlamydia screening without increasing the facilities for screening, further testing for confirmation and for treatment, would cause collapse of the present already overstretched arrangements.
- *Is treatment at an early stage of more benefit than treatment at a later stage?* Definitely – infection can easily be eradicated in the early stages before structural damage occurs. However, it is unknown how often people recover from chlamydial infection without treatment.
- *Are the chances of physical and psychological harm less than the chances of benefit?* This depends on how the test is presented, people's feelings about stigmatisation (having a 'sexually transmitted infection') and public knowledge about the condition.
- *Can the cost be balanced against the benefits the service provides, versus other opportunity costs and benefits?* This is unknown as yet: studies from Merseyside and Southampton showed much higher prevalence of infection and higher costs for the counselling time and number of tests performed than expected.[6,7] The screening is being extended gradually across the UK.

You can read about setting up your own guidelines that might be part of a development plan in your workplace in the book *Sexual Health Matters in Primary Care*.[1]

Managing infection control in general practice

You clear up your swabbing equipment after the patient has left and consider whether you have removed all trace of infection. If you're unsure you could consider using the interactive CD ROM based on the British Medical Association's (BMA's) published guidelines (1998) on blood-borne viruses (HIV, HBV, HCV) that is available from the BMA.[8] Key issues covered include: infection prevention, decontamination methods, safe handling and disposal of sharps, and post-exposure prophylaxis. The Department of Health, Medical Devices Agency and Health and Safety Executive assisted in the development of the material. Your practice team could audit knowledge and procedures before and after its use.

Case study 6.2

The GP refers Miss Pyrexia to the gynaecology ward with lower abdominal pain and a suspected diagnosis of ectopic pregnancy. Her recent menses was 5 days late, lighter than usual and she has an IUD *in situ*. On examination you note she is mildly pyrexial and has mild diffuse lower abdominal tenderness with cervical excitation. You are relieved to find a sensitive pregnancy test is negative and generally she seems well.

Often, it is difficult to establish a conclusive diagnosis of pelvic inflammatory disease (PID) in view of a lack of critical diagnostic criteria. Look at the RCOG guidelines to aid management.[9] A low threshold for prompt treatment is appropriate in view of the risk of long-term tubal damage and worsening severity, so start Miss Pyrexia on antibiotic treatment. Clinical symptoms suggestive of PID include lower abdominal pain and tenderness, deep dyspareunia, abnormal vaginal discharge, cervical excitation and pyrexia (>38°C). Non-specific blood tests that support a diagnosis of PID include raised white cell count, elevated erythrocyte sedimentation rate and elevated C-reactive protein. A pregnancy test and transvaginal ultrasound scan may provide valuable information to exclude alternative pathologies. Test for gonorrhoea and chlamydia in the lower genital tract as described earlier, although it is important to note that absence of lower genital tract infection does not exclude PID.[10,11] A diagnostic laparoscopy may be helpful to exclude alternative pathologies, but it is not without risks. Organisms have been isolated from fallopian tubes that appear normal at laparoscopy.[10,11]

As this patient has only mild PID the IUD may be left *in situ*. The RCOG guidelines concluded that an IUD only increases the risk of developing PID in the first few weeks after insertion and there was no clear benefit for removal in mild PID.[9] Although PID is rare with a viable intrauterine pregnancy, an ectopic pregnancy may present as apparent PID. Do a pregnancy test as part of the routine assessment. Precise details of antibiotic treatment for acute PID varies between hospitals depending on a number of factors including severity of PID, cost, patient preference, local prevalence of infections and antimicrobial sensitivity patterns. The RCOG recommends broad-spectrum antibiotic therapy to cover *N. gonorrhoeae*, *C. trachomatis* and anaerobic infection as detailed in Box 6.2.

Box 6.2:   Antibiotic treatment for PID[9]

In mild or moderate PID (in the absence of a tubo-ovarian abscess), there is no difference in outcome when patients are treated as outpatients or admitted to hospital. Outpatient antibiotic treatment should be based on one of the following regimens:

- oral ofloxacin 400 mg twice a day plus oral metronidazole 400 mg twice a day for 14 days

or

- intramuscular ceftriaxone 250 mg immediately or intramuscular cefoxitin 2 g immediately with oral probenecid 1 g, followed by oral doxycycline 100 mg twice a day plus metronidazole 400 mg twice a day for 14 days.

In more severe cases inpatient antibiotic treatment should be based on intravenous therapy, which should be continued until 24 h after clinical improvement and followed by oral therapy. Recommended regimens are:

- intravenous cefoxitin 2 g three times a day plus intravenous doxycycline 100 mg twice a day (oral doxycycline may be used if tolerated), followed by oral doxycycline 100 mg twice a day plus oral metronidazole 400 mg twice a day for a total of 14 days

or

- intravenous clindamycin 900 mg three times a day plus intravenous gentamicin: 2 mg/kg loading dose followed by 1.5 mg/kg three times a day (a single daily dose of 7 mg/kg may be substituted), followed by either:
  - oral clindamycin 450 mg four times a day to complete 14 days

or

  - oral doxycycline 100 mg twice a day plus oral metronidazole 400 mg twice a day to complete 14 days *or*

- intravenous ofloxacin 400 mg twice a day plus intravenous metronidazole 500 mg three times a day for 14 days

Reproduced with permission from the Royal College of Obstetricians and Gynaecologists *Guideline No. 32 Management of Acute Pelvic Inflammatory Disease* May 2003
www.rcog.org.uk/guidelines.asp?PageID=106

It would be reasonable to treat Miss Pyrexia in an outpatient setting, but arrange a review three days later to ensure improvement and review the results of cultures. A further review one month later provides an opportunity to confirm complete resolution, and if initial cultures were positive then repeat testing may confirm a cure. It is very important to explain to the patient and her partner that they should abstain from intercourse until the completion of treatment as well as explaining the nature of PID with the long-term risks. The patient should be referred with her partner to the GUM clinic for contact tracing and infection screening. If there was a lack of response to oral therapy or a tubo-ovarian abscess on ultrasound scan, then hospital admission would be advisable. In severe cases, surgical treatment may be necessary to divide adhesions and drain pelvic abscesses.

Case study 6.2 continued

Miss Pyrexia feels much better following her course of antibiotics. Aware of the significance of STI she visits the GUM clinic with her partner to pursue contact tracing. In the future, she insists her sexual partner uses condoms as she is keen to reduce the chance of further infection.

Collecting data to demonstrate your learning, competence, performance and standards of service delivery

Example cycle of evidence 6.1

- Focus: research
- Other relevant focus: management

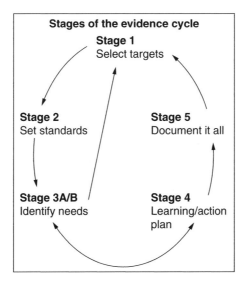

Stages of the evidence cycle

Stage 1
Select targets

Stage 2
Set standards

Stage 5
Document it all

Stage 3A/B
Identify needs

Stage 4
Learning/action plan

Case study 6.3

Dr Leap and Dr Jump are PwSIs in women's health, who want to apply for funding to introduce screening for chlamydia and to be able to offer routine testing for HIV in their practice. They want to be able to show that the service they provide is enhanced by these measures and that the uptake of both services justifies the investment. Their intention is to use a questionnaire to find out the level of knowledge that their service users and staff have, then provide education, information and training as appropriate, so that they can introduce the new services. They will measure the level of knowledge again and the uptake of the new services.

This is just an example. Keep your task simple. You could choose three or four cycles of evidence to demonstrate your competence each year.

Stage 1: Select your aspirations for good practice

The excellent doctor:

- puts the care and safety of patients first when participating in research
- conducts all research in an ethical manner, with honesty and integrity
- is satisfied that in therapeutic research the foreseeable risks will not outweigh the potential benefits to patients
- is satisfied that in non-therapeutic research the potential benefits from the development of treatments and furthering of knowledge far outweigh any foreseeable risks to participants
- completes, if possible, research projects involving patients or volunteers or ensures that they are completed by others (except where harms or risks are expected)
- ensures that care is provided and supervised by staff who have appropriate levels of competence
- ensures that working methods and the working environment conform to health and safety legislation and that safe working practices are followed
- monitors and reviews the quality of the care provided in the work environment.

Stage 2: Set the standards for your outcomes

Outcomes might include:

- the way learning is applied
- a learnt skill
- a protocol
- a strategy that is implemented
- meeting recommended standards.

- Demonstrate consistent best practice in carrying out the research project.
- Demonstrate consistent best practice in the provision of information, teaching and training and service provision regarding the research project.

- Ensure the successful completion of a specific education and training programme by the staff.
- Ensure that all blood products are assumed to be potentially injurious and handled accordingly. A protocol for needle-stick injuries is in place.[9]

Stage 3A: Identify your learning needs

- Find or select a suitable questionnaire to use in an audit of health professionals' knowledge and attitudes about HIV.
- Establish how to write the protocol for the research project and obtain ethical approval. Plan how you will analyse, collate and write up the findings.

Stage 3B: Identify your service needs

> Any of the needs assessment exercises in 3A may also reveal service needs.

- Establish the needs of both staff and patients for information, and of the staff for education and training.
- Manage the changeover from investigating chlamydia to screening for it (*see* Box 6.1).
- Determine how to manage the change to offering HIV testing to all as a routine and the confidentiality issues involved.

Stage 4: Make and carry out a learning and action plan

- Refresh staff research skills and bring them up to date.
- Understand the current requirements for ethical approval.
- Learn more about change management at a workshop.
- Work together to examine the literature and draw up a protocol.
- Read a book or articles about completing research studies.
- Visit other clinics or surgeries already providing these services.

Stage 5: Document your learning, competence, performance and standards of service delivery

- Record the progress with the project as the stages are worked through.
- Write up the project together when complete.
- Re-audit the level of knowledge among staff and patients.
- Include a copy of research ethics approval and permission from the PCO to host the research.
- Include a copy of the evaluation of the project.

Case study 6.3 continued

Dr Leap and Dr Jump quickly abandon the idea of introducing screening for chlamydia because they discover that they would have to wait for funding until their area is eligible. They establish low levels of knowledge among both patients and staff about HIV testing, and after an enthusiastic campaign of information and staff training are able to introduce routine testing for HIV. Their figures show a low level of uptake during the first six months, but a much better uptake by the second six months.

Example cycle of evidence 6.2

- Focus: clinical care
- Other relevant foci: working with colleagues; teaching; probity

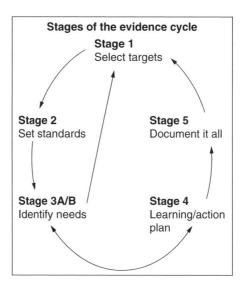

Stages of the evidence cycle

Stage 1
Select targets

Stage 2
Set standards

Stage 5
Document it all

Stage 3A/B
Identify needs

Stage 4
Learning/action plan

Case study 6.4

You are the specialist registrar on call for gynaecology and you are bleeped by your SHO, Dr Failing, to discuss a case. He informs you that he has seen a 38-year-old patient, who he has diagnosed with mild PID as she had severe abdominal pain, dark vaginal bleeding and a pyrexia. The patient had an IUD *in situ* which he has removed, but he did not know which antibiotics to start.

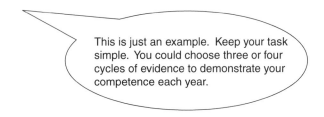

This is just an example. Keep your task simple. You could choose three or four cycles of evidence to demonstrate your competence each year.

Stage 1: Select your aspirations for good practice

The excellent doctor:

- endeavours to ensure patients under his/her care receive safe, appropriate management
- supports colleagues and assists in their education where appropriate
- tells the truth to patients even when mistakes are made.

Stage 2: Set the standards for your outcomes

Outcomes might include:

- the way learning is applied
- a learnt skill
- a protocol
- a strategy that is implemented
- meeting recommended standards.

- Demonstrate consistent best practice in initial assessment and management of patients admitted with lower abdominal pain.
- Ensure junior staff are aware of appropriate management and when to request advice.

Stage 3A: Identify your learning needs

- Review your knowledge of initial assessment and management of patients admitted with lower abdominal pain against referring to national guidelines.
- Ask your junior staff if they feel you have provided them with adequate training in this area.

Stage 3B: Identify your service needs

> Any of the needs assessment exercises in 3A may also reveal service needs.

- Review the local guidelines on the management of patients admitted with lower abdominal pain.
- Audit the number of patients diagnosed with acute PID who have had a pregnancy test checked.
- Review the training junior staff receive on the management of patients admitted with lower abdominal pain including PID.

Stage 4: Make and carry out a learning and action plan

- Compare your knowledge of the initial assessment and management of patients admitted with lower abdominal pain including PID with an authoritative source you obtain and read.
- Prepare a tutorial for the SHOs in your hospital on the initial assessment and management of patients admitted with lower abdominal pain including PID.
- Obtain statistics about the proportion of patients admitted to your hospital with abdominal pain who have PID or ectopic pregnancies.

Stage 5: Document your learning, competence, performance and standards of service delivery

- Include feedback from your SHOs about your training.
- Include the tutorial you give to all the SHOs together with the feedback from them.
- Include the statistics from Stage 4, point 3 above, the results of the audit of pregnancy tests in suspected PID and the action points agreed.

Case study 6.4 continued

When you speak to the SHO on the phone you enquire if a pregnancy test has been performed. As this had not been done, you suggest this is checked while you are on the way to review the patient. When you arrive to see the patient, the SHO is looking red faced as the pregnancy test is positive and the patient's condition has acutely deteriorated. After explaining to the patient that you suspect the initial diagnosis was wrong, you initiate immediate resuscitation for the patient and shortly later in theatre remove a ruptured ectopic pregnancy. Tactfully you discuss the difficulty of the diagnosis of ectopic pregnancy.

You mention it is a sensible precaution to perform a pregnancy test on any woman suspected as having PID, as an ectopic pregnancy has a notoriously variable presentation. You arrange a tutorial for all SHOs to discuss management of acute abdominal pain. During this tutorial, you cover many issues including that an IUD may be left *in situ* in women with clinically mild PID but should be removed in cases of severe disease.

References

1 Wakley G and Chambers R (2002) *Sexual Health Matters in Primary Care.* Radcliffe Medical Press, Oxford.

2 The most recently available statistics on STIs are available from www.hpa.org.uk

3 Adler MW (1999) *ABC of Sexually Transmitted Diseases.* BMJ Publishing Group, London.

4 Godlee F (ed.) (2004) *Clinical Evidence Concise.* BMJ Publishing Group, London. www.clinicalevidence.com

5 Joint Formulary Committee (2004) *British National Formulary.* British Medical Association and Royal Pharmaceutical Society of Great Britain, London. www.bnf.org

6 Harvey J, Webb A and Mallinson H (2000) *Chlamydia trachomatis* screening in young people in Merseyside. *Journal of Family Planning and Reproductive Health Care.* **26:** 199–201.

7 Basarab A, Browning D, Lanham S and O'Connell S (2002) Pilot study to assess the presence of chlamydia trachomatis in urine from 18–30-year-old males using EIA/IF and PCR. *Journal of Family Planning and Reproductive Health Care.* **28:** 36–7.

8 Board of Science and Education, British Medical Association (1998) *Bloodborne Viruses and Infection Control: a guide for health care professionals.* Interactive CD ROM. BMJ Books, London.

9 Royal College of Obstetricians and Gynaecologists (2003) Guideline No. 32 *Management of Acute Pelvic Inflammatory Disease.* www.rcog.org.uk/guidelines. asp?PageID=106

10 Bevan CD, Johal BJ, Mumtaz G *et al.* (1995) Clinical, laparoscopic and microbiological findings in acute salpingitis: report on a United Kingdom cohort. *British Journal of Obstetrics and Gynaecology.* **102:** 407–14.

11 Morcos R, Frost N, Hnat M *et al.* (1993) Laparoscopic versus clinical diagnosis of acute pelvic inflammatory disease. *Journal of Reproductive Medicine.* **38:** 53–6.

Further reading

- Avert (UK based charity giving extensive AIDS information). www. avert.org
- Carter Y, Moss C and Weyman A (eds) (2004) *RCGP Handbook of Sexual Health in Primary Care* (2e). Royal College of General Practitioners, London.
- Department of Health National Strategy for Sexual Health and HIV. www.dh.gov.uk/assetRoot/04/06/22/64/04062264.pdf
- Genitourinary infections and GUM clinic list (British Association for Sexual Health and HIV). www.bashh.org
- *Guidelines* – summarising clinical guidelines for primary care (latest issue). Representatives of professional bodies and organisations producing guidelines. Medendium Group Publishing Ltd, Berkhamsted. www.eguidelines. co.uk This gives the source for the full guidelines for any particular condition.
- STI Online includes issues of *Sexually Transmitted Infections* published since 1967 and includes *Genitourinary Medicine* and *British Journal of Venereal Diseases.* http://sti.bmjjournals.com
- Scottish Intercollegiate Guidelines Network (SIGN). www.sign.ac.uk
- Members of the BMA Foundation for AIDS (2002) *Take the HIV Test.* Published by Medical Foundation for AIDS and Sexual Health, BMA House, Tavistock Square, London WC1H 9JP. www.medfash.org.uk
- Wakley G, Cunnion M and Chambers R (2003) *Improving Sexual Health Advice.* Radcliffe Medical Press, Oxford.

7

Infertility

At least one in six couples are referred to secondary care for infertility management.[1] Infertility occupies a substantial component of a gynaecological service, with increasing rates of referral due to improvements in treatment that have attracted media attention. Postal questionnaires dividing infertility into primary infertility, where the couple have never achieved a pregnancy, and secondary infertility, where they have previously achieved a pregnancy, suggested that around 16% of couples experience primary infertility after one year and 9% of couples after two years.[2,3] These studies suggested a further 16% of couples experience secondary infertility after one year and 5% of couples after two years. Not all couples reach secondary care, with at least one in four couples reporting infertility at some time,[2] and the true scale of infertility may be even greater due to under-reporting in replies to questionnaires.

An infertility consultation takes longer than a standard gynaecological consultation as you usually need to take a history and perform examinations for both a man and a woman, issues are often complex to explain and the couple are frequently distressed. Results of initial assessments are usually required to establish a management plan. In many cases, these are arranged before the initial visit but even then they may be incomplete. It may be wise at the start of the consultation to explain what you will cover and arrange a further visit to establish a definitive management plan when all the results are to hand. At the initial consultation, the first priority is to provide some prognostic information reassuring the couple that although infertility is common, most couples will ultimately achieve a pregnancy. Secondly, it is important to take this opportunity for pre-pregnancy assessment to optimise the outlook for a healthy pregnancy and normal baby. Specific assessment regarding infertility should be commenced in a systematic fashion.

In order to manage infertile couples it is important to have a basic understanding of this subject. The British Fertility Society in collaboration with the RCOG has developed a special interest training programme in general infertility (*see* Box 7.1). This chapter provides a helpful overview and references for further reading.

Box 7.1:   Syllabus of the British Fertility Society and Royal College of
Obstetricians and Gynaecologists for special skills training in infertility[4]

1   The epidemiology of infertility
2   Initial assessment of the infertile couple
3   Male factor infertility
4   Disorders of ovulation
5   Tubal factor infertility
6   Infertility and endometriosis
7   Unexplained infertility
8   Psychological aspects of reproductive medicine
9   Ultrasound skills
10 *In vitro* fertilisation (IVF) and other assisted reproduction techniques
11 Epidemiology, research, statistics and audit
12 Teaching
13 Ethical and legal aspects
14 Administration

Case study 7.1

Mrs Brie, a 32-year-old woman, together with her 43-year-old husband, is
referred to your clinic as they are concerned that they have not achieved a
pregnancy after trying for 12 months. Mrs Brie is a hairdresser with a passion
for soft cheeses and her husband is a sheep farmer, who has been pleased with
the expansion of his farm in the last few years. Mrs Brie had a miscarriage three
years earlier which they found very distressing and it has taken them some
time to decide to try for a further pregnancy. Mr Brie is a healthy farmer keen to
have an heir to take over the farm when he retires.

   Mrs Brie has read on the internet that dietary changes can have a major
impact on fertility. You suspect Mrs Brie's passion for food may extend beyond
soft cheese as she weighs 80 kg at a height of 1.6 m (body mass index 31 kg/m^2).
Her menstrual cycle is regular at 28 days' duration and she notices mid-cycle
abdominal discomfort when her cervical mucus also seems more profuse.

What issues you should cover

Even before reviewing test results, it is possible to give the couple useful
prognostic information by considering their age, duration of infertility and any
prior pregnancies.[2] Although it may be tempting to reassure the couple that
12 months is too soon to worry, it is important to establish how long the couple

have been having intercourse without contraception. Couples may stop contraception without actively trying for a pregnancy and only regard the period of infertility as the time that they were actively trying for pregnancy. Although fertility declines with female age, the outlook remains good at 32 years. The influence of male age is much less marked. As the couple have achieved a pregnancy in the past, they are more likely to achieve a further pregnancy, even though the previous pregnancy did not lead to a baby.

The couple may find it useful for you to give them some idea of the average time to conception based on their circumstances. It is possible to calculate this from Tables 7.1 and 7.2 or use the fertility calculators on the website: www.repromed.org.uk/book/content/Fertility_Calculator.htm.

Such calculators only provide a guide, and individual circumstances may alter the prognosis. In this case, Mrs Brie is obese which may have an adverse influence even though she appears to be ovulating. She certainly should be encouraged to lose weight, setting realistic targets for weight loss.

Table 7.1: A guide to prognosis for pregnancy without fertility treatment: average baseline prognosis[5]

Months	Cumulative live-birth rate (%)
3	13.0
6	18.9
12	27.4
24	41.9
36	46.2

Table 7.2: A guide to prognosis for pregnancy without fertility treatment: effects of prognostic factors[5]

Effects of prognostic factors (if result of postcoital test is available)		Effects of prognostic factors (if no postcoital test is performed)	
Prognostic factor	Multiplication factor	Prognostic factor	Multiplication factor
Duration of infertility <24 months	1.5	Prior pregnancy in partnership	1.5
Ovulation defect	0.4	Duration of infertility <24 months	1.5
Abnormal PCT	0.3	Female age <30 years	1.4
Tubal defect	0.1	Male defect (WHO)	0.6
		Ovulation defect	0.4
		Tubal defect	0.1

Mrs Brie has particular risks from toxoplasmosis from the sheep and listeria from soft cheeses. An important aspect of infertility management is to give general lifestyle advice including about smoking, alcohol intake, occupational risks and diet. It is important to explain risks without causing undue alarm and suggest simple measures such as, in this case, avoidance of soft cheeses, and the sheep, particularly at lambing time.

From a study based on 726 couples in primary care, a prognostic model for spontaneous conception has been developed.[5] Despite cynicism leading many not to perform the postcoital test (PCT), the study showed the PCT had such a powerful prognostic effect that two versions of the model had to be constructed. The baseline cumulative pregnancy rate is modified by applying each multiplication factor that applies to the couple, providing an individual-ised chance of pregnancy. For instance if a couple's duration of infertility is <24 months, multiplying the baseline rate by 1.5 would give their increased cumulative live-birth rate. If a couple had a duration of infertility of <24 months and had a tubal defect, then the baseline rate would be multiplied by 1.5 times 0.1.

NICE released a comprehensive set of guidelines regarding the management of infertile couples including initial assessment and lifestyle advice.[6] Although the full guidelines may be a little daunting to work through, the summary document and management flow charts are a useful source of information for initial management. Pre-pregnancy tests include rubella immunity and rou-tine cervical cytology. Pre-pregnancy advice covers areas such as stopping smoking, reducing alcohol, optimising weight and taking folate to reduce risk of neural tube defects. Ovulation is assessed by progesterone on day 21 of a 28-day cycle or later if the cycle is longer. Serum follicle stimulating hormone (FSH) and luteinising hormone (LH) at the start of the menstrual cycle can provide further useful information. A basic semen analysis is the first step in male investigations.

Unexplained infertility

In many cases, initial assessment may uncover no specific cause for infertility. Even after comprehensive assessment, at least one in four couples' infertility may be classified as 'unexplained' (see Table 7.3).

Table 7.3: Relative percentages of major diagnostic categories in three series of infertile couples

	Netherlands[5] (n = 726) (%)	Canada[7] (n = 2198) (%)	UK[1] (n = 708) (%)
All male factor	30	27	26
Azoospermia	5	7	6
Ovulatory	26	27	21
Tubal	13	26	14
Endometriosis	3	14	6
Unexplained	30	26	28

Note that as couples may have more than one cause for infertility the total proportions exceed 100%.

Case study 7.1 continued

Mr and Mrs Brie return to your surgery with the results of their initial investigations. Although initially following the miscarriage the couple had used condoms, they had stopped using any contraception over 14 months previously. Mrs Brie has joined a local dieting club and since you last saw her six weeks previously she has lost 3 kg in weight. She has found this very difficult to achieve and wonders if any treatment could help her to lose further weight. At this stage, there is no clear pointer to the cause of infertility, but optimisation of her weight is likely to improve her chances of achieving a spontaneous conception.

It is important to provide the couple with reassurance and support, explaining the likelihood of conception if they persevere. As the couple have over one year's infertility, it is reasonable to refer to them to the local fertility clinic, particularly if the waiting list is long, as this secures their place in the 'queue' to be seen.

Weight reduction will not only benefit the chance of achieving a pregnancy but also will also improve the outlook for any pregnancy and have wider health benefits. The National electronic Library for Health provides guidance on weight reduction, including the place for medications and surgery.[8]

In many cases there are multiple infertility factors often affecting both the male and female side. It is always important to manage a couple together and plan management that considers all factors. If you have access to hysterosalpingography, this can provide very valuable information.

> **Case study 7.2**
>
> Mr and Mrs Fallow attend your surgery to discuss their infertility tests that you had arranged when they had consulted you earlier, following 18 months of infertility at the ages of 37 and 39 years respectively. Although recent chlamydia swabs had been negative, in the past Mrs Fallow had been treated for a bout of serious PID. In view of the risk of tubal disease, you arranged a hysterosalpingogram that revealed large bilateral hydrosalpinges. Her chlamydia serology is strongly positive but her other test results are unremarkable. Mr Fallow's external genitalia appear normal on examination and semen analysis is: volume 2.5 ml, pH 7.4, concentration 14 million per ml, motility 40% normal, morphology 4% normal forms.

Although hysterosalpingograms may suggest a tube is blocked when it is not in around 10% of cases, they are reliable at identifying hydrosalpinges. The prognosis for tubal surgery in this case is likely to be poor partly because of the unfavourable factors of large hydrosalpinges and chlamydia serology and because of the poor semen result (*see* Box 7.2 for normal values). Although the low borderline sperm count and reduced motility are of uncertain significance, the poor morphology suggests a poor prognosis. If these results were confirmed with a repeat semen test, the optimal treatment would be assisted conception using intracytoplasmic sperm injection (ICSI).

It is known that large hydrosalpinges reduce pregnancy rates and increase miscarriage rates. Thus salpingectomy, or at least occlusion of the proximal fallopian tubes, should be considered before proceeding with ICSI. The couple need referral for specialist care and, if they proceed with ICSI treatment, they will need to be tested for hepatitis B and C and HIV to comply with the Human Fertilisation and Embryology Authority's (HFEA's) guidelines on the storage of sperm and embryos.[9]

Box 7.2: World Health Organization normal semen analysis values[10]

- Volume 2 ml or more
- pH 7.2 or more
- Sperm concentration >20 million per ml
- Total sperm number 40 or more million sperm per ejaculate
- Motility >50%
- Morphology 15% or more normal forms
- Sperm antibody tests
  - immunobead test <50% motile sperm bound to beads
  - mixed agglutination reaction (MAR) test <50% motile sperm bound to beads

Male factor infertility

Around one in four infertile couples have evidence of male factor problems, and around one in 20 show a complete absence of any sperm. It is vital to know how to manage the couple following the semen result particularly as they may become very distressed and even angry if the news is bad.

Case study 7.3

Mr and Mrs Baron have completed basic infertility investigations and have arranged an appointment with you to review their results. Mrs Baron has a cousin who has cystic fibrosis but she is a healthy 31 year old with no known medical problems. Mr Baron takes a beta-blocker for hypertension, which is well controlled and he is otherwise well. The results of the investigations are given below.

Mrs Baron

- Rubella antibodies detected confirming immunity
- LH 3.1 IU/l FSH 4 IU/l
- Progesterone 38 nmol/l
- Chlamydia serology negative

Mr Baron: semen analysis

- Volume 3.2 ml
- pH 7.2
- Liquefaction: normal
- No sperm were observed

At the initial consultation, you had not examined Mr Baron, but in view of the above discovery you now examine him. You discover that his testicles are small and he has a moderate-sized varicocele on the left hand side. You are unable to positively identify his vas deferens on either side.

The main priority of the male genitalia examination is to identify lumps that could be testicular cancer and that necessitate urgent referral. Checking for small testicular volumes and the absence of the vas deferens can provide very helpful information. If you are unfamiliar with this examination then it may be worth arranging to sit in on a clinic with a local specialist to learn more. There are conflicting views on the importance of varicoceles in male infertility, but the treatment of varicoceles is unlikely to be beneficial if the sperm count is very low.

Drugs may affect sperm production and/or ability to achieve intravaginal ejaculation. If you encounter such a problem with a man on medication, consider a causal relationship. As a first step, consult the *British National Formulary (BNF)*[11] and seek expert opinion if this does not provide an answer.

Azoospermia may be caused by chromosome abnormalities, hence it is advisable to check his karyotype and also screen for Y deletions. The azoospermia could be caused by congenital bilateral absence of the vas deferens, which is associated with the carriage of cystic fibrosis mutations. In view of this genetic risk to the child, it is important to screen the couple for carriage of cystic fibrosis mutations and arrange genetic counselling if appropriate.

The treatment options open to the couple are donor insemination or surgical sperm retrieval followed by ICSI. Both treatments are effective, with pregnancy rates of 30% for one cycle of ICSI or about three cycles of donor insemination. Where there is an obstructive cause for azoospermia, it is usually possible to collect sperm surgically, although if there are primary testicular problems then in many cases no sperm may be collected. A low testicular volume, a high serum FSH level and, possibly in the future, a low serum inhibin B level may help predict the risk of failure to collect sperm surgically.

Ovulatory infertility

Irregular menstruation is a useful pointer to ovulatory dysfunction, which may be very responsive to appropriate treatment. However, to clarify the cause of irregular periods further tests are required beyond the basic investigations (*see* Table 7.4).

Case study 7.4

Mr and Mrs Nimble are a young couple who have completed basic infertility investigations. Mrs Nimble is a slim aerobics instructor who has erratic, extremely painful periods occurring at anything from 4 to 10 week intervals. Her sister was recently diagnosed with endometriosis so Mrs Nimble is very concerned about her painful menses. In view of this, you had arranged a few additional tests:

- LH 14 IU/l
- FSH 4 IU/l
- thyroid stimulating hormone (TSH) 2 nmol/l
- prolactin 240 mU/l
- SHBG 20 nmol/l
- testosterone 3.2 nmol/l

The most common cause for irregular menstruation is PCOS. This case has the typical biochemical features of a raised LH, raised LH/FSH ratio (above 2.5),

Table 7.4: Tests that may be helpful when ovulatory dysfunction is suspected

Test	
FSH and LH	It is important to ensure that FSH and LH are measured at the start of the menstrual cycle. If measured later in the cycle there is a risk that these test results will be elevated due to the mid-cycle surge of both LH and FSH. The FSH and LH serum levels may be suppressed, if taking hormones such as the combined oral contraceptive pill. Levels vary from month to month and the highest result is the most important. High FSH levels are suggestive of diminished fertility and ovarian failure. High LH levels are associated with polycystic ovary syndrome (PCOS), particularly if the woman has an irregular menstrual cycle with hirsutism. Low levels of both FSH and LH are seen with hypothalamic underactivity, which can cause absent menses (amenorrhoea).
Progesterone	To provide a guide as to whether ovulation has occurred, progesterone needs to be measured around 7 days prior to menstruation, on day 21 of a 28-day cycle. Even in fertile women, ovulation will not occur in all cycles so a single low result should not cause immediate concern and it may be repeated. Even when ovulation does occur, the progesterone rise may not always be great and even if progesterone is high, this does not always mean that an oocyte has been released from the ovary.
Prolactin	Raised prolactin levels (hyperprolactinaemia) are associated with ovulatory dysfunction, oligomenorrhoea, amenorrhoea and galactorrhoea. Hyperprolactinaemia is induced by many causes including certain drugs (e.g. phenothiazines), but when there is no obvious cause it is usually due to a small (<2 mm) tumour that is secreting excess prolactin in the pituitary gland. However, it is important to visualise the pituitary gland to exclude a larger pituitary tumour as this could press on the optic nerves impairing vision.
Thyroid function tests	Thyroid dysfunction may disturb the menstrual cycle and it is beneficial for pregnancy to achieve a euthyroid status prior to fertility treatment.
Androgens (e.g. testosterone) and sex hormone binding globulin (SHBG)	High androgens are most commonly associated with PCOS. It is important to also measure SHBG when assessing androgen levels. If the SHBG level is low, the free androgen level may be high even if the total androgen level is normal.

raised testosterone and lower SHBG levels. However, in many patients this is not the case and expert opinion is divided on the precise definition of PCOS, including the role and appearance of ultrasonography of the ovaries. Although hyperprolactinaemia is an infrequent cause of irregular menstruation, it is important to check prolactin levels, as one of the causes is pituitary tumours.

The first step in the management of anovulatory PCOS is weight reduction if the woman is obese, but, as with this patient, not everyone with PCOS is obese.

Opinion is divided regarding initial medication. First-line treatment used to be anti-oestrogen therapy with clomiphene, but concerns about the risk of multiple pregnancies and ovarian cancer now make this approach less attractive. Insulin-sensitising agents such as metformin are used increasingly.

Particularly as this patient is concerned about endometriosis, laparoscopy may assist management. Laparoscopy is the best way to assess the pelvis and provides the opportunity for therapy to ablate any endometriosis and to diathermy the ovaries, if anti-oestrogen and metformin therapy prove unsuccessful. Although the mechanism of action of ovarian diathermy remains unclear, it has been shown to be as effective in PCOS as is using gonadotrophins for ovulation induction. Although medical treatment for endometriosis has not been shown to improve infertility, some studies have suggested a benefit from surgical ablation. It is important to discuss such treatment options with the patient prior to the laparoscopy, explaining the potential risks of diathermy.

Collecting data to demonstrate your learning, competence, performance and standards of service delivery

Example cycle of evidence 7.1

- Focus: clinical care
- Other relevant focus: confidentiality

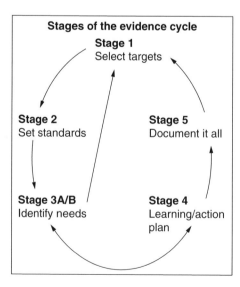

> **Case study 7.5**
>
> Mrs Noble visits the gynaecology clinic at the start of her period to have a blood test for FSH and LH by your clinic nurse for infertility assessment. She asks the clinic nurse if the result of her husband's semen test is available yet. She has read an article on the internet suggesting that she could improve her fertility by altering her diet. Your clinic nurse discovers the semen test revealed a complete absence of sperm and bleeps you to ask what she should say to Mrs Noble.
>
> As it would be a breach of confidentiality in respect of Mr Noble to give his wife his semen test result, you discuss the confidentiality issues with your clinic nurse. Your clinic nurse agrees that the results should be conveyed personally to Mr Noble with due sensitivity.
>
> You recall the management plan was for the *couple* to return for a follow-up consultation to discuss the results when they are all available. Accordingly, you ask the clinic nurse to check that such an appointment has been made and defer any discussion of results until then.

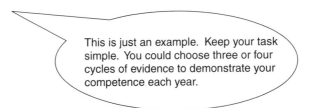

This is just an example. Keep your task simple. You could choose three or four cycles of evidence to demonstrate your competence each year.

Stage 1: Select your aspirations for good practice

The excellent doctor:

- keeps comprehensive records outlining the management plan and information given to patients including details of how results will be followed up and patients informed of results
- ensures that information is conveyed sensitively and appropriately respecting confidentiality.

Stage 2: Set the standards for your outcomes

Outcomes might include:

- the way learning is applied
- a learnt skill
- a protocol
- a strategy that is implemented
- meeting recommended standards.

- Demonstrate consistent best practice in providing assessment and treatment for infertile couples. Check the last 10 couples to establish that each had completed the basic tests outlined in RCOG guidelines.[5]
- Demonstrate consistent best practice in keeping good patient medical records, for instance by auditing the 10 consultation records to see if the management plan was recorded at the end of each consultation.

Stage 3A: Identify your learning needs

- Consider if you know how to interpret the semen results that come from your local service, particularly considering what information you need to give to a patient depending on the result and what actions you should take.
- When recording data such as a semen analysis, undertake an audit that the notes incorporate a check to review whether action is required such as checking that the patient has an appointment to discuss the result.
- Reflect on whether you know the current views on the link between diet and infertility.

Stage 3B: Identify your service needs

> Any of the needs assessment exercises in 3A may also reveal service needs.

- Track what happens to basic semen reports when received by the practice.
- Check whether the local laboratory follows WHO guidelines and that the results they produce are consistent with WHO normal values.[10]
- Discuss with practice staff what information they give to patients about results of sensitive tests such as semen analysis.

Stage 4: Make and carry out a learning and action plan

- Read about semen tests, causes of abnormality and subsequent management options.
- Write up a simple handout for patients going through the significance of the results of the infertility tests you arrange, and discuss this with colleagues.
- Meet with the practice staff to talk through aspects of confidentiality of medical records. Consider producing (or updating) confidentiality guidelines for staff including reference to relevant resources such as:
  - www.dataprotection.gov.uk
  - www.gmc-uk.org

Stage 5: Document your learning, competence, performance and standards of service delivery

- Keep track of all infertility consultations over a year and review how the patients were assessed and informed of results.
- Discuss your approach to infertility with other health professionals and obtain their feedback.
- File your patient infertility results information sheet in your portfolio.

Case study 7.5 continued

Mr and Mrs Noble return to your clinic two weeks later, by which time you have had time to refresh yourself on the management of azoospermia and obtain all the test results. The couple are relieved that you gave them this news together and had a clear plan of action, starting with a repeat semen test for confirmation of the results. Having heard this news, they are less interested in the role of diet in infertility but are pleased that you are aware of the subject providing them with simple advice and reassurance.

Example cycle of evidence 7.2

- Focus: maintaining good medical practice

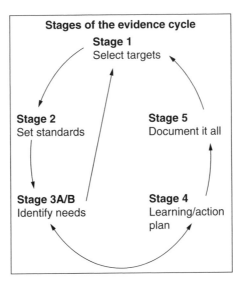

Stages of the evidence cycle

Stage 1
Select targets

Stage 2
Set standards

Stage 5
Document it all

Stage 3A/B
Identify needs

Stage 4
Learning/action plan

Case study 7.6

Mrs Jumble presents to the clinic with irregular menstruation and for a repeat prescription of 'infertility tablets' (clomiphene). Although she has been taking these for six months, her menstrual cycle remains irregular. Her mother had ovarian cancer and she has concerns that she may develop cancer herself. You notice she is a little overweight and perhaps slightly hirsute. She had been told that she has PCOS and she wonders if she could try a better treatment.

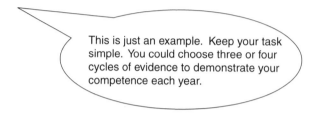

This is just an example. Keep your task simple. You could choose three or four cycles of evidence to demonstrate your competence each year.

Stage 1: Select your aspirations for good practice

The excellent doctor:

- knows where to find best evidence on practice
- completes prescribing audits at routine intervals to ensure that patients do not continue treatment inappropriately.

Stage 2: Set the standards for your outcomes

Outcomes might include:

- the way learning is applied
- a learnt skill
- a protocol
- a strategy that is implemented
- meeting recommended standards.

- Demonstrate knowledge about best practice for the initial treatment options for ovulation induction in PCOS.
- Demonstrate best practice in the management of patients with PCOS.

Stage 3A: Identify your learning needs

- Discuss best current practice in the provision of insulin-sensitising agents, such as metformin, for treatment in PCOS with the appropriate specialist consultant. Realise some of what you didn't know previously.

Stage 3B: Identify your service needs

Any of the needs assessment exercises in 3A may also reveal service needs.

- Audit the use of clomiphene in the clinic and consider whether it has been monitored adequately and whether metformin may be a better alternative.
- Discuss the guidelines for the management of patients with infertility problems with relevant staff, to determine whether any amendments are required.

Stage 4: Make and carry out a learning and action plan

- Perform a literature search for recent recommendations, especially any systematic reviews, for current best practice for treatment in PCOS.
- Obtain relevant guidelines e.g. from the RCOG. In this case, the RCOG provides useful guidelines on infertility,[12] the National electronic Library for Health provides access to Cochrane systematic reviews,[8] and the *British National Formulary* gives details about drugs.[11] These resources will suggest metformin is regarded as an effective treatment for PCOS and that long-term use of clomiphene may increase the risk of developing ovarian cancer. Additional advice will include the importance of losing weight and the small risk of lactic acidosis should the patient take metformin.

Stage 5: Document your learning, competence, performance and standards of service delivery

- Incorporate the new information in the guidelines for the use in your practice by all the clinicians.
- Record the results of your literature search regarding evidence-based guidelines in Stage 4 above.
- Re-audit the management of PCOS to confirm that the modern management guidelines are being followed.

Case study 7.6 continued

Mrs Jumble presents three months later delighted that her menstrual cycle is now regular and she is optimistic that she may become pregnant.

Example cycle of evidence 7.3

- Focus: relationships with patients

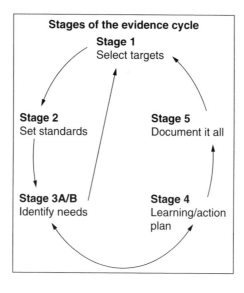

Case study 7.7

Mr and Mrs Lament attend your surgery to discuss their infertility tests. The hysterosalpingogram has revealed large bilateral hydrosalpinges and her husband has a low sperm count. You start to explain that they have serious barriers to a pregnancy and they may require assisted conception treatment. Mr Lament enquires whether there is anything he can do to improve his fertility. Mrs Lament wonders why she has developed tubal problems when she was never aware of any pelvic infection in the past. As the consultation progresses and you start to explain that it may be advisable to remove the fallopian tubes before considering assisted conception treatment Mrs Lament starts to cry.

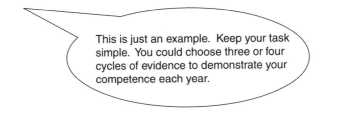

This is just an example. Keep your task simple. You could choose three or four cycles of evidence to demonstrate your competence each year.

Stage 1: Select your aspirations for good practice

The excellent doctor:

- provides patients with sufficient information to make choices about their management
- provides support for patients faced with difficult decisions and frustrations.

Stage 2: Set the standards for your outcomes

Outcomes might include:

- the way learning is applied
- a learnt skill
- a protocol
- a strategy that is implemented
- meeting recommended standards.

- Demonstrate best practice in providing information to patients.
- Develop your counselling skills through appropriate courses or through mentorship with a suitable peer or senior colleague.

Stage 3A: Identify your learning needs

- Self-assess your learning needs about breaking bad news – after an occasion when you had to do that.
- Complete a quiz or multiple choice questionnaire on a website or GP newspaper about interpretation of results of infertility tests.

Stage 3B: Identify your service needs

Any of the needs assessment exercises in 3A may also reveal service needs.

- Get feedback from colleagues and staff for whom you are responsible, as to whether you recognise and are sensitive to patients' feelings and have strategies to deal with distressed patients.
- Take part in a 360° feedback exercise arranged by the practice team – focusing on breaking bad news and enabling patients to make informed decisions about treatment.

Stage 4: Make and carry out a learning and action plan

- Ask a colleague who has done a breaking bad news course to facilitate role-play scenarios of difficult patient–staff interactions, where the patient is very distressed, at an in-house educational session for the team.
- Attend a course on breaking bad news.
- Sit in a clinic on one or more occasions with an infertility specialist and ask a myriad of questions about infertility tests and treatment.

Stage 5: Document your learning, competence, performance and standards of service delivery

- Keep records of interactions with other distressed patients and record your conclusions about your improvement in your reflective diary.
- Make notes from your attendance at the course.
- Keep copies of feedback from others in the team.

Case study 7.7 continued

You feel that you have identified the need for time in dealing with infertile couples when breaking bad news, and will consider how best to handle this in your surgery.

Example cycle of evidence 7.4

- Focus: working with colleagues
- Other relevant focus: teaching and training

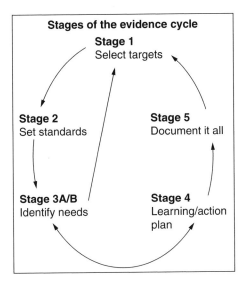

Stages of the evidence cycle

Stage 1
Select targets

Stage 2
Set standards

Stage 5
Document it all

Stage 3A/B
Identify needs

Stage 4
Learning/action plan

Case study 7.8

A medical student is sitting in your clinic when a patient arrives asking for advice for infertility. The GP referral letter mentions that she has had a milky discharge from her breasts and has had no periods for four months.

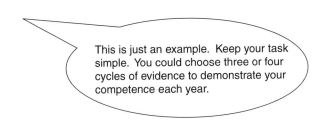

This is just an example. Keep your task simple. You could choose three or four cycles of evidence to demonstrate your competence each year.

Stage 1: Select your aspirations for good practice

The excellent doctor:

- helps to educate other colleagues at all levels
- does not undermine the confidence of juniors or students.

Stage 2: Set the standards for your outcomes

Outcomes might include:

- the way learning is applied
- a learnt skill
- a protocol
- a strategy that is implemented
- meeting recommended standards.

- Demonstrate an active involvement in the training of another.
- Consider your standard for 'working with colleagues'.

Stage 3A: Identify your learning needs

- Obtain peer review of your teaching skills: ask another trainer to peer review your tutorial with the medical student.
- Self-assess your awareness of the curriculum of the local medical school.
- Check that your knowledge about galactorrhoea and amenorrhoea are up to date by comparing your performance with best practice guidelines.
- Feedback from trainees is a good way to assess your teaching (although it may be difficult to avoid bias, if feedback is not anonymised).
- Check whether you can answer questions posed by the medical student and whether you have the skills to guide the student to solve clinical problems, while taking care to ensure that the patient understands what he says.

Stage 3B: Identify your service needs

Any of the needs assessment exercises in 3A may also reveal service needs.

- Undertake a force-field analysis with others in the practice team about the driving and restraining factors involved in practice-teaching medical students.

Stage 4: Make and carry out a learning and action plan

- Attend a meeting of the medical school curriculum group and ask for details of their relevant policies for 'working with colleagues' including such specifics as dress code, consenting patients to be seen and possibly examined by medical students.

- Attend an update meeting about galactorrhoea and amenorrhoea and read widely about these subjects to increase your knowledge in this area.
- Attend a 'Training the trainers' course or, if it is a while since you last went on a course, a refresher may be a good idea.
- Reflect on the outcome of the force-field analysis with other teachers in the practice. Make a plan to boost driving factors.

Stage 5: Document your learning, competence, performance and standards of service delivery

- Keep the feedback from the medical student.
- Record the outcome of the force-field analysis and your reflections.
- Include your downloaded notes about galactorrhoea.
- Keep a copy of the completed quiz with the corrected answers where relevant.

Case study 7.8 continued

At the end of the consultation, the patient feels happy that her condition has been explained so thoroughly and feels confident that a knowledgeable doctor is managing her. The medical student is grateful for the opportunity to learn about galactorrhoea and amenorrhoea with a real clinical perspective.

Summary

This chapter has provided an introduction to the management of the infertile couple and there are many texts that provide more details.[13,14] Although infertility is a common problem, the majority of infertile couples will achieve their desire to have a child. Whereas past studies have suggested that 3–7% of couples never achieve this goal,[2,3] recent advances in treatment will reduce this figure further. In the next chapter, the management of assisted conception couples will be considered where this is appropriate. Issues of healthcare economics, ethics, patient choice and awareness of options will play a major role in how many couples remain involuntarily childless. NICE released guidance in early 2004 on the 'assessment and treatment for people with fertility problems' in the National Health Service,[6] and there appears to be overwhelming public support to end the current inequalities of access to IVF throughout the UK (*see* Box 7.3).

Box 7.3:   The public's views about funding of infertility treatment

The science and discovery centre, At-Bristol and the Centre for Reproductive Medicine, University of Bristol surveyed visitors to the central shopping centre in Bristol and to the science centre website. Over 800 members of the public revealed overwhelming support for NHS funding of infertility services and an end to the 'postcode lottery' of funding for this provision. The survey showed that it was not generally felt that treatment should be denied solely due to a lower chance of success. However, the age of the mother was an important consideration with different views on what the upper age limit should be. In February 2004 NICE produced guidance on the provision of NHS funded infertility treatment that it is hoped may lead to more consistent treatment throughout the NHS.[15]

References

1   Hull MG, Glazener CM, Kelly NJ et al. (1985) Population study of causes, treatment, and outcome of infertility. British Medical Journal. **291:** 1693–7.

2   Gunnell DJ and Ewings P (1994) Infertility prevalence, needs assessment and purchasing. Journal of Public Health Medicine. **16:** 29–35.

3   Templeton A, Fraser C and Thompson B (1990) The epidemiology of infertility in Aberdeen. British Medical Journal. **301:** 148–52.

4   www.fertility.org.uk/education/

5   Snick HK, Snick TS, Evers JL and Collins JA (1997) The spontaneous pregnancy prognosis in untreated subfertile couples: the Walcheren primary care study. Human Reproduction. **12:** 1582–8.

6   NICE (2004) Fertility: assessment and treatment for people with fertility problems. http://www.nice.org.uk/page.aspx?o=104435

7   Collins JA, Burrows EA and Willan AR (1995) The prognosis for live birth among untreated infertile couples. Fertility and Sterility. **64:** 22–8.

8   www.nelh.nhs.uk

9   Human Fertilisation and Embryology Authority (2001) Screening of Patients. Letter 6th June 2001 from HFEA chairman to all IVF clinics. HFEA, London.

10   World Health Organization (1999) WHO Laboratory Manual for the Examination of Human Semen and Sperm-Cervical Mucus Interaction (4e). Cambridge University Press, Cambridge.

11   www.bnf.org

12   www.RCOG.org.uk

13 Cahill DJ and Wardle PG (2002) Management of infertility. *British Medical Journal.* **325:** 28–32. http://bmj.com/cgi/content/full/325/7354/28?maxto show=

14 Jenkins JM, Corrigan L and Chambers R (2002) *Infertility Matters in Healthcare.* Radcliffe Medical Press, Oxford.

15 www.bionews.org.uk/commentary.lasso?storyid=1719

8

Assisted reproduction

Since the birth of Louise Brown in 1978, assisted conception has seen incredible changes (*see* Box 8.1). More than a million babies have been born following assisted conception worldwide. Although the UK has a relatively low provision of assisted conception compared to the rest of Europe, over 1 in 100 babies born in the UK in 2000 were conceived by IVF. In February 2004, NICE released guidelines that require a massive expansion in IVF services so these figures are likely to rise.[1] The British Fertility Society, in collaboration with the RCOG, has developed a special interest training programme in assisted reproduction (*see* Box 8.2). This chapter will provide an overview of assisted reproduction with references for further reading. Although this chapter is written from the perspective of a practitioner, it is important to appreciate the patient's perspective. Amidst what sometimes is a highly complex treatment schedule, patients may feel very vulnerable, disempowered and desperate to have a child. One way to appreciate this depth of feeling is to visit one of the infertility patients' online discussion forums and see what they are saying.[2]

Box 8.1:   Historical dates

- First test tube baby: July 1978
- First frozen embryo birth: 1983
- First surrogate baby: January 1985
- First embryo screening for anomaly: 1988
- First baby born following sperm injection into egg: 1990
- Surgical sperm retrieval: 1993
- First 'frozen egg' baby: 1997

Box 8.2:   Syllabus of British Fertility Society and Royal College of Obstetricians and Gynaecologists for special skills training in assisted reproduction[3]

1   Basic skills in the management of the infertile
2   Patient selection for IVF
3   Controlled ovarian stimulation
4   Oocyte retrieval

5   Ultrasound skills in assisted reproduction techniques (ART)
6   Embryology
7   Embryo transfer
8   Implantation
9   Gamete donation
10 Psychological aspects of reproductive medicine
11 Epidemiology, research, statistics and audit
12 Teaching . . .
13 Ethical and legal aspects

Case study 8.1

You notice that the last couple in your clinic have a thick set of notes detailing a long history of infertility including tubal surgery 18 months earlier. The semen analysis seems to have been suboptimal to you, and the couple are both aged 37 years. When the couple come in to see you, they tell you that they wish to have assisted conception treatment and having surfed the internet they have many questions to ask.

What issues you should cover

Patient selection for IVF

When considering assisted conception, further assessment is required to select the appropriate treatment options, which are outlined in Table 8.1. Often there is a choice of treatments, thus it is important to counsel patients regarding the pros and cons of each option to involve them in the final decision. For instance, when to use intracytoplasmic sperm injection (ICSI) or donor insemination (DI) is very much a personal decision for the couple to make. Short-term and long-term risks to patients and their offspring should be discussed.[4] Generally, research to date is reassuring. For instance, data from 114 628 IVF cycles reveal that emergency admissions to hospital following IVF occur infrequently – ovarian hyperstimulation syndrome 0.9%, bleeding 0.07% and infection 0.03%.[5] The majority of patients who persevere with IVF treatment will ultimately have at least one child. The chance of a live birth is over 25% per treatment cycle below 35 years of age, but falls to less than 10% beyond 40 years age. The chance of success in individual couples is greatest in the first few cycles then gradually declines. Overall, around 90% of IVF pregnancies

Table 8.1:   Assisted conception treatment options and indications

Treatment type	Indications
IVF: although this literally means fertilisation 'in glass', in practice fertilisation takes place outside the body in a plastic container	• Tubal infertility • Unexplained infertility • Where other treatments have proven unsuccessful such as ovulation induction and donor insemination
ICSI: a single sperm is injected into the egg to enable fertilisation with very low sperm counts or other problems such as low motility	• Male factor problems e.g. low sperm count, low sperm motility, high percentage abnormal sperm morphology, significant anti-sperm antibodies • Previous low or failed fertilisation with IVF

Surgical sperm recovery (SSR): collection of sperm by various surgical methods when no sperm is present in the ejaculate	• Obstructive azoospermia e.g.
	  – failed vasectomy reversal
	  – cystic fibrosis
	• Testicular failure

DI: artificial insemination with donor sperm that has been stored frozen following careful screening	• For patients who choose not to have ICSI when they have a major sperm problem or where it is not possible to obtain viable sperm even following surgical sperm retrieval • Male genetic disorders to avoid the risk of transmission of a gene to a child or where no viable sperm are produced
Donor eggs (DE): eggs are donated by one woman for the treatment of another using IVF. (Egg sharing refers to when a patient having IVF uses some eggs for herself and donates the rest of the eggs to another patient usually in return for a reduction in her treatment costs)	• Premature ovarian failure • To avoid risk of transmitting female genetic disorders • Gonadal dysgenesis • Oophorectomy • Ovarian failure after chemotherapy/radiotherapy • Selected cases of IVF treatment failures (for example poor response)
Gamete intrafallopian tube transfer (GIFT): eggs are collected from ovaries then at laparoscopy placed in fallopian tubes with prepared sperm	• This treatment was used for unexplained infertility particularly when IVF was unavailable • With increasing availability and successfulness of IVF, the place of GIFT has reduced substantially

Endometriosis is not a specific indication for assisted conception unless associated with prolonged infertility and/or the presence of tubal damage and pelvic adhesions.

occur in the first four attempts. It is important to quote local pregnancy rates as results vary between centres.[6]

Patients need a prognostication of their chances of a live birth with treatment, which should reflect not only national data but also local audit of success. Female age is one of the greatest predictors of success, but it is important to explain the concept of biological age where women's fertility declines at different rates so that some women may become menopausal in their 20s whereas others may have a child naturally in their late 40s. The serum FSH provides a crude measure of the female biological age (*see* Figure 8.1). However, the FSH value is only a crude indicator and it does not exclude the possibility that the ovaries may respond poorly, particularly as the patient becomes older. Box 8.3 indicates several other factors that influence prognosis and the presence of hydrosalpinges deserves particular mention. Significant hydrosalpinges both reduce the chance of implantation and increase the risk of miscarriage. Although salpingectomy prior to IVF has been shown to improve outcome, other more conservative approaches such as proximal occlusion of the fallopian tubes are favoured by many, encouraging more research into optimal management.[7]

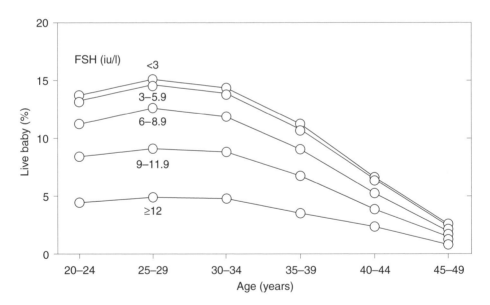

Figure 8.1:   Mathematical model illustrating the probability of a live baby arising from a single embryo transferred for different bands of age and basal serum FSH based on a study of the first IVF/ICSI cycle of 1019 couples.[8]

Box 8.3: Factors that affect the outcome of IVF treatment

Good prognosis

- Young age (*see* Figure 8.1)
- Previous pregnancy
- Previous successful fertility treatment

Poor prognosis

- Older age (*see* Figure 8.1)
- Long duration of infertility
- Previous failed fertility treatment
- Obesity (body mass index >30)
- Smoking (active and passive)
- Untreated hydrosalpinx
- Basal serum FSH levels >10 IU
- Poor response to ovarian stimulation

Controlled ovarian stimulation

In the natural cycle, the primordial ovarian follicles go through a prolonged period of growth probably lasting several months and unrelated to menstruation. Most follicles never reach full maturity and become atretic. It is generally felt that women are born with a certain number of oocytes that decline with age, although recently this has been challenged with the discovery of possible stem cells in mice ovaries.[9] Each month, a number of follicles start the process of completing their development under the action of FSH, with a permissive influence from LH. Both FSH and LH are glycoproteins released from the pituitary in response to pulsatile stimulation by gonadotrophin releasing hormone (GnRH) from the hypothalamus. In humans, each month usually only one follicle becomes dominant and a single oocyte is released following a surge of LH triggered by rising oestradiol levels produced by the dominant follicle. By giving women FSH injections, it is possible to prevent follicle dominance and recruit multiple mature follicles so that more oocytes may be available for collection. However, the rising oestradiol levels from the multiple follicles produced may prematurely trigger a LH surge. To prevent this premature trigger, GnRH analogues are usually administered as part of a controlled ovarian stimulation regime. The analogues may be either agonists that initially stimulate then suppress FSH/LH release, or antagonists that directly suppress FSH/LH release. The final maturation of the follicle is triggered by an injection of human chorionic gonadotrophin (HCG), which acts on a common receptor to LH. When an analogue has been used, luteal support may be beneficial usually in the form of progesterone pessaries or injections.

Over time, gonadotrophin preparations have developed from initially impure, highly variable urine-derived products to later much more pure urinary products and even now genetically engineered recombinant products.[10] The relative efficacy of these products is disputed but all appear to be effective. Other issues favouring recombinant products are now drawing further consideration such as theoretical safety issues surrounding infective agents such as prions, more precise methods of measuring the amount of drug in commercial formulations to reduce batch-to-batch variation, and ease of patient use with improved delivery systems such as 'gonadotrophin pens'.

Monitoring of controlled ovarian stimulation is best achieved with experienced transvaginal ultrasonography. Serum oestradiol levels may be helpful to confirm poor response when it difficult to be sure if there is really no follicular development. Serum oestradiol levels may also be helpful when there are concerns of potential over-response. It has become common practice in many centres to withhold FSH stimulation when oestradiol levels become too high, and defer HCG injections until levels fall to an acceptable level (coasting). Both poor response and over-response to gonadotrophins, leading potentially to ovarian hyperstimulation syndrome, are major issues.

Ovarian hyperstimulation syndrome (OHSS) is the most clinically significant short-term morbidity following ovarian stimulation with gonadotrophins. Despite extensive research, complete prevention is not as yet possible, with significant OHSS complicating about 1 in 20 IVF cycles, although it presents a serious problem in only a small number of cases.[11] Patients may present with lower abdominal discomfort, bloating, and nausea that may progress to vomiting and in severe cases ascites, pleural effusion and even thromboembolic disease. The pathophysiology is poorly understood and management is mainly supportive. Hospitalisation may be necessary for observation, pain relief, antiemetics, intravenous fluids and thromboprophylaxis. A high haematocrit is a useful guide to severity, and attention to fluid balance is important. OHSS is difficult to predict though it is more common with PCOS particularly in younger patients. Improved management of gonadotrophin stimulation appears to have reduced OHSS, but vigilance remains important with referral for expert advice when OHSS is suspected.

Oocyte retrieval

Oocyte retrieval is usually scheduled around 34 to 38 h after the administration of HCG. If the procedure is too early, the oocytes may not be sufficiently mature and may be difficult to collect. If the procedure is too late, the oocytes may have been spontaneously released from the ovary. Oocyte retrieval is conducted in an operating theatre that may be quite small, but care must be taken to provide a clean environment to reduce the risk of infection. Not everyone uses antibiotics routinely, but they may be helpful in at-risk situations such as puncture of an endometrioma. Usually the procedure is conducted under transvaginal ultrasound control with the patient having an empty bladder, although other approaches, including laparoscopic and transvesical, are possible. Anaesthesia is required as the procedure can be painful for patients. This varies from local anaesthetic with analgesics, to 'conscious sedation' to light general anaesthetic. Although 'conscious sedation' may be painful at the time, it has been argued because of the amnesic effect of the drugs used, that patients do not recall the pain. This is the method endorsed by the NICE infertility guidelines.[1] However, others challenge the ethics of this approach and point to patients who subsequently become aware of the suppressed painful episode developing manifestations such as night terrors.

The immediate complications of oocyte retrieval include perforation of a viscus and haemorrhage. Fortunately, the probability of inadvertent perforation of a viscus with good technique is very low. Most ultrasound machines provide a visual guide to the path of the needle to ensure this enters directly into the ovary on first puncture, and throughout the procedure it is important to maintain sight of the tip of the needle. Some haemorrhage at the puncture site within the vagina may commonly occur, but this can usually be controlled by firm direct pressure for at least 5 min, and suturing is rarely required.

Ultrasound skills in ART

It is essential for clinicians to have a sound grasp of both the physics and practice of ultrasonography. In particular, it is important to be able to appreciate normal and abnormal pelvic anatomy and make accurate measurements of ovarian follicles and endometrial thickness. Early pregnancy scanning is also very important to include identification of the site, viability and gestation of the pregnancy paying attention to the possibility of heterotopic pregnancies following multiple embryo transfer.

Gamete donation

Gamete donation is a complex area including donation of sperms, oocytes, embryos and surrogacy. The organisation of services is complex, particularly where this involves the recruitment and screening of donors. Appropriate patient selection and counselling is essential with particular attention paid to the welfare of the child and relevant legislation.[12]

Donor insemination is usually performed in a natural cycle, initially using cervical insemination but progressing to intra-uterine insemination if this proves unsuccessful. A single insemination is usually sufficient and may be timed by the menstrual cycle guided by cervical mucus changes and LH dipsticks where necessary.

Oocyte and embryo donation are more complex, requiring IVF on the part of the donor and preparation of the uterus of the recipient, usually by hormone-regulated cycles using oestrogen and progesterone with suppression of endogenous hormones using a GnRH analogue where necessary.

Surrogacy may be technically simple where the host is inseminated by the male patient's sperm, or more complex where the couple's embryo obtained by IVF is replaced into the host's uterus primed by a hormone-regulated cycle. In either case, there are complex ethical and legal issues to consider, including the risk that either the host or the couple may change their mind following birth, leaving the child in a fraught situation.

Embryology

Although clinicians may not be expected to perform laboratory procedures, a basic understanding of embryology will assist clinical practice. A good approach is to first read relevant textbooks,[13,14] and the local laboratory protocol manual then spend some time in the laboratory with an experienced scientist to observe practical procedures.

Embryo transfer

There are a variety of different embryo transfer catheters which are often chosen by personal preference rather than objective evidence of superiority. Key differences include two-piece after-loading design, soft atraumatic tips, degree of flexibility, visibility on ultrasound and tip design. With a two-piece catheter, the outer part of the catheter may be introduced into the uterus and only when this has been achieved are the embryos introduced using an inner catheter that slides through the outer catheter. This greatly reduces the stress of what can be a very anxious time for the patient and also the operator, who may initially struggle to insert the catheter. An atraumatic tip with a flexible catheter sounds attractive, but the cervical canal has multiple blind-ending crypts into which such a catheter can enter complicating the procedure and causing bleeding. This is particularly a problem when the cervical canal is acutely curved from anteflexion or retroflexion. It has been suggested that ultrasound guidance may improve the transfer procedure, although this does not distinguish whether any benefit relates to visualising the catheter, or to the full bladder that is necessary to use the ultrasound and straightens the cervical canal thus simplifying the transfer procedure. Further tip design may be even more important with the bulb tip seen on some catheters enabling them to pass over the cervical crypt openings and safely navigate the cervical canal to the uterus. It is generally agreed that the tip of the embryo catheter must pass above the internal cervical os but should avoid hitting the fundus of the uterus.

Where transfer is particularly difficult then sedation may be administered to overcome discomfort, and if it is not possible to pass through the cervix then the embryos may be inserted directly into the uterine cavity using a trans-myometrial needle.

The greatest risk of assisted conception is multiple pregnancy, in view of the likelihood of problems later in the pregnancy, particularly prematurity. This is why the HFEA limits IVF treatment to the transfer of no more than two embryos other than in exceptional circumstances. Patients can be reassured that limiting the number of embryos replaced in high-quality centres reduces multiple pregnancy significantly, without making a big impact on pregnancy rates (*see* Table 8.2). There is an increasing move within the profession to transfer a single embryo in suitable patients, although, understandably, patients who are paying for treatment are reluctant to accept this option.

Table 8.2: Pregnancy rates at the Centre for Reproductive Medicine prior to the move to routine two-embryo transfer where at least four embryos were available for transfer (January 1997 to December 2000)[15]

Age	Two embryos transferred			Three embryos transferred		
	Pregnancy rate %	Twins %	Triplets %	Pregnancy rate %	Twins %	Triplets %
<35 years	33.4 (n=311)	25	2.9	31.7 (n=432)	35	13.9
35–39 years	25.5 (n=94)	12.5	0	29.9 (n=347)	31.7	4.8
≥40 years	25 (n=12)	67	0	15 (n=113)	17.6	0

Implantation

The physiology of implantation in the human is incompletely understood but may be vulnerable to a number of areas including local endometrial regulatory factors, factors released by the embryo and possible immunological influences.

The potential of the embryo may be the most critical factor as ectopic pregnancies in relatively inhospitable sites are well recognised.

Psychological aspects of reproductive medicine

The importance of psychological factors cannot be over-emphasised when dealing with an infertile couple. It was always well recognised that extremes of stress may lead to amenorrhoea. Although during an IVF cycle psychological factors may be overcome by the powerful medication used, the stress to both men and women can be extreme, reaching levels of psychiatric depression and anxiety. This can lead to failure of men to produce a sperm sample when required on the day of oocyte retrieval, and cause grief to the couple. Following an unsuccessful cycle patients may be particularly vulnerable and support counselling is an integral part of management. Long-term psychosexual disorders may result from infertility and these should be actively sought and managed even if the couples decide against further fertility treatment. If patients are aware of what they may experience during treatment, this may lessen their stress. Good patient information is an essential component of management covering not only the details of the treatment but also what side-effects they may experience (*see* Box 8.4).

Box 8.4:   Patient side-effects during IVF treatment

- Most patients experience hot flushes and possibly mild headaches while taking GnRH agonists that finish when oestradiol levels rise as gonadotrophin stimulation starts. Some patients experience a range of other side-effects such as mood swings and irritability.
- The menstrual period at the start of the IVF cycle may be prolonged with occasional spotting, again until the oestradiol levels rise.
- During gonadotrophin stimulation patients may experience pelvic discomfort as the ovaries enlarge.
- Following the oocyte retrieval there is usually some pain, worse initially but possibly continuing over a few days varying from mild discomfort to potentially significant pain. Reassure patients they will have the pain relief they individually require to ensure they are comfortable.
- Embryo transfer is usually no more uncomfortable than having a cervical smear.
- Following the oocyte retrieval, the most important side-effects to look out for are related to OHSS including abdominal pain unrelieved by analgesia, abdominal bloating, nausea and vomiting. Patients should be advised to seek medical advice if they experience these symptoms.

Epidemiology, research, statistics and audit

Epidemiological research is required to determine the long-term risks to both patients and their offspring. Despite theoretical concerns that controlled ovarian hyperstimulation with gonadotrophins may increase the risk of malignancy, the balance of evidence is reassuring that this treatment does not increase the lifetime risks of either gynaecological or breast cancer, beyond the increased risks known for infertile women compared to fertile women.[16,17] Although the vast majority of children conceived by assisted conception appear normal in all respects, a higher proportion of these children have abnormalities when compared with natural conceptions.[18,19] This is mainly due to the increased age of infertile patients presenting for treatment, increased risks with multiple pregnancies and subtle gene defects in either partner, or poor reproductive function in general, but a treatment effect cannot be excluded. Counsel patients appropriately particularly with regard to the advantages of limiting the number of embryos replaced.

Although anything to do with statistics fills many with dread, approached in small bite size pieces most can come to grips with a working knowledge of statistics. The *British Medical Journal* provides an excellent starter book freely available online: *Statistics at Square One*.[20]

The HFEA website provides useful guidance on ethical and legal aspects of assisted conception practice.[12]

Collecting data to demonstrate your learning, competence, performance and standards of service delivery

Example cycle of evidence 8.1

- Focus: clinical care
- Other relevant focus: oocyte retrieval

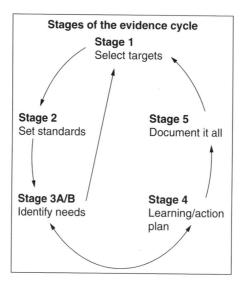

Stages of the evidence cycle

Stage 1
Select targets

Stage 2
Set standards

Stage 5
Document it all

Stage 3A/B
Identify needs

Stage 4
Learning/action plan

Case study 8.2

Over the course of a year, you wish to develop your skills in transvaginal oocyte retrieval. You wish to become an independent practitioner with this skill, able to deal with all suitable cases.

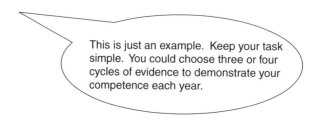

This is just an example. Keep your task simple. You could choose three or four cycles of evidence to demonstrate your competence each year.

Stage 1: Select your aspirations for good practice

The excellent doctor:

- understands how to operate the equipment he/she uses
- is able to perform tasks independently to an appropriate level of proficiency compared to his/her peers
- performs ongoing audit to demonstrate a satisfactory level of proficiency.

Stage 2: Set the standards for your outcomes

Outcomes might include:

- the way learning is applied
- a learnt skill
- a protocol
- a strategy that is implemented
- meeting recommended standards.

- Perform at least 75 oocyte retrievals as principal operator with at least half of these as sole operator.
- Achieve independent competent proficiency in transvaginal oocyte retrieval.
- Aim to collect the same average number of oocytes as the experienced staff within the same centre within the same average time.

Stage 3A: Identify your learning needs

- Self-assess your knowledge of the equipment used and seek guidance from a senior colleague to fill any gaps. Make sure you are aware of the steps taken to set up the equipment including equipment sterilisation procedures, ensuring the ultrasound machine has the correct settings, choice of needle, calibration of the pump pressure and sterile technique.
- You need to feel self-confident about your proficiency in transvaginal ultrasonography before you attempt to use a needle for transvaginal oocyte retrieval. You should practise scanning patients during ovarian stimulation to become competent in three-dimensional orientation of the ultrasound probe and be able to identify the needle tip on the screen while your mentor is performing the oocyte retrieval.

Stage 3B: Identify your service needs

> Any of the needs assessment exercises in 3A may also reveal service needs.

- Establish how many oocyte retrievals are performed in your unit and how many you would be able to perform. Particularly in NHS units there may be limits imposed on the number of oocyte retrievals, due to financial constraints.
- Check how much time is allocated to the theatre list and ensure there will be sufficient time for your training on the list. See if this is consistent with experience in other centres.

Stage 4: Make and carry out a learning and action plan

- Ensure you have a suitably experienced, appropriately qualified trainer(s) who will train you how to perform this procedure. Ideally your trainer should be recognised as a preceptor by the British Fertility Society (BFS)/ RCOG.
- If necessary, arrange basic ultrasound training and use of equipment before proceeding to oocyte retrievals by attending a teaching workshop followed by in-house training with a log book.
- Initially observe oocyte retrievals by your trainer, then your trainer will collect oocytes from the first ovary and you collect oocytes from the second ovary; later collect oocytes from both ovaries under direct supervision and finally collect oocytes without direct supervision but with your trainer available if required. As your confidence builds you will be able to perform oocyte retrievals on more complex cases.
- Ensure you are able to meet the service needs of the centre. If necessary arrange a unit meeting to review workload, timing, efficiency of theatre bookings, etc.
- To set your targets, audit the average number of oocytes collected and the average time taken by experienced staff.

Stage 5: Document your learning, competence, performance and standards of service delivery

- Record the number of oocytes you collect against the number of follicles on scan, the duration of the oocyte retrieval procedure and any complications. Plot this on a chart for each 10 consecutive cases you complete against the target set from Stage 4 above.

- Ultimately seek the signature of your trainer to confirm you are independently competent in oocyte retrievals.

Case study 8.2 continued

Ultimately you achieve competence in this technique and perform lists on your own, while your trainer is seeing patients in the nearby IVF clinic.

Example cycle of evidence 8.2

- Focus: teaching and training
- Other relevant focus: working with colleagues

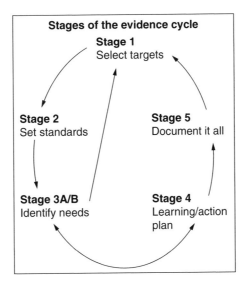

Stages of the evidence cycle

Stage 1
Select targets

Stage 2
Set standards

Stage 5
Document it all

Stage 3A/B
Identify needs

Stage 4
Learning/action plan

Case study 8.3

The lecturer who covers the undergraduate lectures on reproductive physiology in the male and female is going on maternity leave in four months' time. You are requested to stand in for the lecturer to provide these lectures.

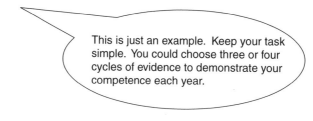

This is just an example. Keep your task simple. You could choose three or four cycles of evidence to demonstrate your competence each year.

Stage 1: Select your aspirations for good practice

The excellent doctor in relationships with colleagues:

- is supportive of other team members when there are difficulties with health, conduct or performance but not to the detriment of patients
- makes suitable arrangements for the continuation of all professional responsibilities.

And in teaching and training:

- contributes to the education of students or colleagues willingly
- develops the skills, attitudes and practices of a competent teacher if he/she has responsibilities for teaching
- ensures that students and junior colleagues are properly supervised in line with the responsibilities he/she has for teaching them.

Stage 2: Set the standards for your outcomes

Outcomes might include:

- the way learning is applied
- a learnt skill
- a protocol
- a strategy that is implemented
- meeting recommended standards.

- Be able to relay appropriate information regarding female and male reproductive physiology to students of reproductive health. Deliver two lectures covering these topics including aspects of clinical relevance.
- Ensure that your lectures fit in with the other lectures delivered. Have a clear timetable for who is delivering which lecture, covering what details, and when and where the lecture will be delivered and to whom.

Stage 3A: Identify your learning needs

- Self-assess your teaching and training skills e.g. reflect on your teaching experience and skills, or seek a suitable local course.
- Review written materials from previous lectures: peer discussion to give you more insights into the appropriateness of the lectures with regard to the needs of the students.
- Ask a senior colleague both to discuss the planning of the lectures and observe you deliver them to check that the knowledge and skills you are imparting are up to date and best practice.

Stage 3B: Identify your service needs

> Any of the needs assessment exercises in 3A may also reveal service needs.

- Find out about the requirements of the syllabus regarding reproductive physiology.
- Discuss with your mentor in your unit not only this specific teaching need but also how your teaching skills in general may be developed.
- In discussion with the team and senior consultant, establish if there are any other service needs arising from the maternity locum where you may be able to help.

Stage 4: Make and carry out a learning and action plan

- Attend a refresher course on teaching and training.
- Write, and obtain feedback from a senior colleague on, training materials for the topic.
- Read widely about the subject of the reproductive physiology – *see* references at the end of this chapter and seek advice from a senior colleague.

Stage 5: Document your learning, competence, performance and standards of service delivery

- Complete a weekly diary sheet of duties illustrating additional duties undertaken to relieve colleagues of duties arising from redistribution of tasks in connection with the maternity locum.
- Log the feedback on your teaching, training and written materials.
- Record your teaching notes and student feedback.

Case study 8.3 continued

The lectures you develop prove very popular with the medical students. You develop a sound understanding of reproductive physiology with improvements in your teaching skills.

Example cycle of evidence 8.3

- Focus: working with colleagues on ethical issues

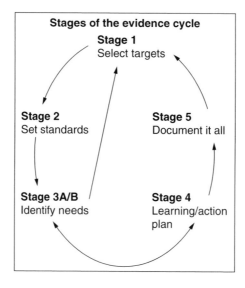

Case study 8.4

A 49-year-old Nigerian woman requests donor oocyte treatment having secured the agreement of her 34-year-old sister to provide donated oocytes. Her sister's husband is against this suggestion, but her sister wishes to do all she can to help, aware that it may be difficult to find a suitable altruistic egg donor. The case has been referred to the centre's ethics committee for advice and you have been invited to attend as part of your training.

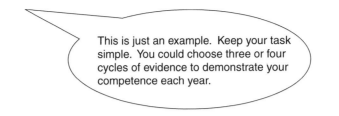

This is just an example. Keep your task simple. You could choose three or four cycles of evidence to demonstrate your competence each year.

Stage 1: Select your aspirations for good practice

The excellent doctor in relationships with colleagues:

- respects the views of colleagues and is prepared to change his/her mind in the light of new information
- communicates his/her opinion clearly and fully even about complex issues.

Stage 2: Set the standards for your outcomes

Outcomes might include:

- the way learning is applied
- a learnt skill
- a protocol
- a strategy that is implemented
- meeting recommended standards.

- Understand the relevant laws governing use of donor gametes.
- Understand the constitution and operation of the ethics committee.

Stage 3A: Identify your learning needs

- Self-assess the extent to which you understand the principles of ethical review (beneficence, non-maleficence, autonomy, justice) and how they could apply to assisted conception treatment.[21]
- Discuss what is meant by the 'welfare of the child' in the HFE Act 1990, with a well informed colleague with special interest in ethical issues, to check if your understanding is correct.[22]

Stage 3B: Identify your service needs

Any of the needs assessment exercises in 3A may also reveal service needs.

- Check on the availability of donor oocytes including the availability for different racial groups in your unit. Compare your findings with those for similar units if possible.
- Enquire about the methods of donor recruitment used in your unit and investigate the options to purchase donor gametes from elsewhere (a search on the internet may provide you with a number of options).
- Consider the service provision in other centres in respect of their ethical review process and general attitudes regarding donor gametes.[23]

Stage 4: Make and carry out a learning and action plan

- Attend a lecture on ethics of donor gamete treatment.
- Review the current HFEA code of conduct.[24]
- Document the issues to consider for a tutorial with a member of the centre's ethics committee.

Stage 5: Document your learning, competence, performance and standards of service delivery

- Log the whole ethical process but take care to respect the confidentiality of the patients ensuring that you do not mention their names in your record.

Case study 8.4 continued

After lengthy deliberation the ethics committee recommends that the request for treatment should not be supported despite their sympathy for the couple. There were reservations on the age of the patient to become a mother. However, the main concern related to the inevitable pressure on the sister to donate the oocytes, which may force her to donate oocytes even if she was unsure this was appropriate. This could lead to a complex situation for the child, whose rights must be respected. Following further discussion the senior IVF staff inform the couple with due sensitivity that treatment will not be provided, but that counselling support is available.

References

1. NICE (2004) Fertility: assessment and treatment for people with fertility problems. www.nice.org.uk/page.aspx?o=104435

2. www.ReproMED.co.uk/forum

3. www.fertility.org.uk/education

4. Land JA and Evers JLH (2003) Risks and complications in assisted reproduction techniques: Report of an ESHRE consensus meeting. *Human Reproduction.* **18:** 455–7.

5. Nygren KG and Nyboe Andersen A (2002) Assisted reproductive technology in Europe, 1999. Results generated from European registers by ESHRE. *Human Reproduction.* **17:** 3260–74.

6. Dobson R (2002) Data on IVF clinics show wide variation in success rate. *British Medical Journal.* **325:** 460.

7. Hammadieh N, Afnan M, Evans J *et al.* (2004) A postal survey of hydrosalpinx management prior to IVF in the United Kingdom. *Human Reproduction.* **19:** 1009–12.

8. Akande VA, Fleming CF, Hunt LP, Keay SD and Jenkins JM (2002) Biological versus chronological ageing of oocytes, distinguishable by raised FSH levels in relation to the success of IVF treatment. *Human Reproduction.* **17:** 2003–8.

9. Johnson J, Canning J, Kaneko T *et al.* (2004) Germline stem cells and follicular renewal in the postnatal mammalian ovary. *Nature.* **428:** 145–50.

10. Gleicher N, Vietzke M and Vidalil A (2003) Bye-bye urinary gonadotrophins? Recombinant FSH: a real progress in ovulation induction and IVF? *Human Reproduction.* **18:** 476–82.

11. Aboulghar MA and Mansour RT (2003) Ovarian hyperstimulation syndrome: classifications and critical analysis of preventive measures. *Human Reproduction Update.* **9:** 275–89.

12. www.hfea.gov.uk

13. Johnson MH and Everett BJ (1999) *Essential Reproduction* (5e). Blackwell Science Ltd, London.

14. Elder K and Dale B (2000) *In vitro Fertilisation* (2e). Cambridge University Press, Cambridge.

15. www.ReproMED.co.uk

16. Venn A, Watson L, Lumley J *et al.* (1995) Breast and ovarian cancer incidence after infertility and in vitro fertilisation. *Lancet.* **14:** 995–1000.

17. Kashyap S, Moher D, Fung MK *et al.* (2004) Assisted reproductive technology and the incidence of ovarian cancer: a meta-analysis. *Obstetrics and Gynecology.* **103:** 785–94.

18   Helmerhorst FM, Perquin DAM, Donker D *et al.* (2004) Perinatal outcome of singletons and twins after assisted conception: a systematic review of controlled studies. *British Medical Journal.* **328:** 261.

19   Kurinczuk JJ (2003) Safety issues in assisted reproduction technology. *Human Reproduction.* **18:** 925–31.

20   http://bmj.bmjjournals.com/statsbk

21   Stern JE, Cramer CP, Green RM *et al.* (2003) Determining access to assisted reproductive technology: reactions of clinic directors to ethically complex case scenarios. *Human Reproduction.* **18:** 1343–52.

22   HMSO (1990) *Human Fertilisation and Embryology Act 1990* (c.37). www.hmso. gov.uk/acts/acts1990/Ukpga_19900037_en_1.htm

23   ESHRE Task Force on Ethics and Law (2002) III. Gamete and embryo donation. *Human Reproduction.* **17:** 1407–8.

24   HFEA (2004) *Sixth Edition of the HFEA Code of Practice.* HFEA, London. www. hfea.gov.uk/HFEAPublications/CodeofPractice

9

Vaginal bleeding problems

Many vaginal bleeding problems may lead a woman to seek medical advice both in primary and secondary care. This chapter focuses on some of the more common bleeding problems related to menstruation and early pregnancy and provides references to more in-depth information.

Menorrhagia

Case study 9.1

Mrs Flud is a 43-year-old woman, who you are asked to see in view of your special interest in women's health. Over the last five months the patient's periods have become increasingly heavy and troublesome. Her menstrual cycle remains regular and she had a normal cervical smear six months earlier. She feels tired all the time and fed up with her heavy periods. However, she does not want a hysterectomy and she is concerned that if she seeks medical help from the hospital she will be forced to lose her uterus.

What issues you should cover

Before considering treatment, it is important to consider whether there may be any significant underlying pathology. The RCOG provides helpful guidelines on the initial management of menorrhagia, summarised in Figure 9.1. The full guidelines may be viewed by visiting the RCOG website.[1] If following examination, you find that Mrs Flud has no obvious worrying features you can next consider treatment options.

A study of a cohort of women in Oxford up to the end of 1989 suggested that around one in five women in the UK had had a hysterectomy before 55 years of age.[2] In many of these cases the uterus was normal, particularly in parous women. However, improvements in conservative management of menorrhagia provide many options to improve Mrs Flud's heavy periods without a hysterectomy,[3] and the RCOG provides guidelines for medical management in

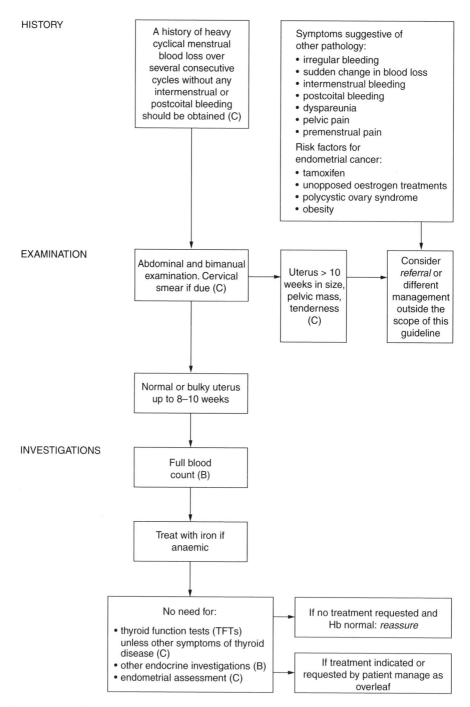

HISTORY

A history of heavy cyclical menstrual blood loss over several consecutive cycles without any intermenstrual or postcoital bleeding should be obtained (C)

Symptoms suggestive of other pathology:
- irregular bleeding
- sudden change in blood loss
- intermenstrual bleeding
- postcoital bleeding
- dyspareunia
- pelvic pain
- premenstrual pain

Risk factors for endometrial cancer:
- tamoxifen
- unopposed oestrogen treatments
- polycystic ovary syndrome
- obesity

EXAMINATION

Abdominal and bimanual examination. Cervical smear if due (C)

Uterus > 10 weeks in size, pelvic mass, tenderness (C)

Consider *referral* or different management outside the scope of this guideline

Normal or bulky uterus up to 8–10 weeks

INVESTIGATIONS

Full blood count (B)

Treat with iron if anaemic

No need for:
- thyroid function tests (TFTs) unless other symptoms of thyroid disease (C)
- other endocrine investigations (B)
- endometrial assessment (C)

If no treatment requested and Hb normal: *reassure*

If treatment indicated or requested by patient manage as overleaf

Figure 9.1: Clinical evaluation of the complaint of menorrhagia (reproduced with permission from the Royal College of Obstetricians and Gynaecologists).[1] Level of evidence: (A), based on randomised controlled trials; (B), based on other robust experimental or observational studies; (C), based on more limited evidence but the advice relies on expert opinion and has the endorsement of respected authorities.

primary care (*see* Figure 9.2). The levonorgestrel IUS is a good method that has been shown to produce up to a 90% reduction in menstrual loss.[4] The IUS also

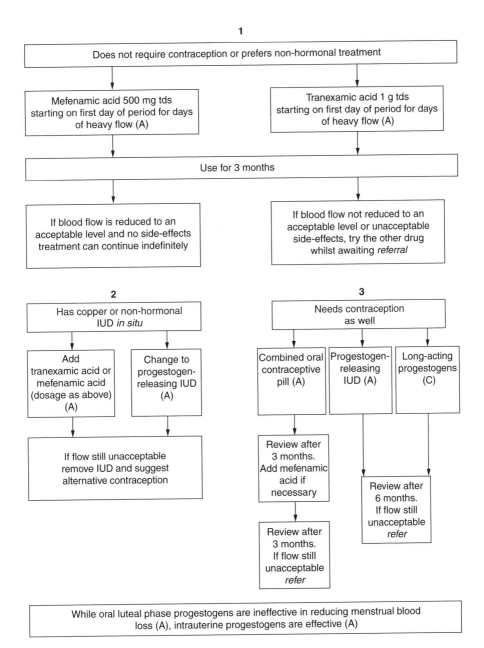

Figure 9.2: Medical management of menorrhagia (reproduced with permission from the Royal College of Obstetricians and Gynaecologists).[1] This figure outlines different approaches to treatment depending on whether the patient does not require contraception (1), is using non-hormonal contraception (2) or requires contraception (3). Evidence levels (A), (B) and (C) are the same as in Figure 9.1.

reduces dysmenorrhoea and provides contraception[4] (*see* Chapter 5 for further details).[5]

Even if medical therapy is unsuccessful, there are several new techniques to ablate the endometrium without removing the uterus, producing satisfactory results in 80–90% of patients.[6] Check on local availability and gynaecologists' experience with new techniques such as balloon systems delivering local heat in the uterus, devices delivering radiofrequency thermal energy or electromagnetic energy in the uterine cavity and endometrial cryoablation. Even if Mrs Flud has symptomatic fibroids, uterine artery embolisation conserving the uterus has been suggested to provide a satisfactory result in the majority of cases.[7]

Case study 9.1 continued

Mrs Flud has no indicators of serious pathology but a full blood count shows that she is mildly iron deficient and she starts taking some oral iron. After discussion of the options, she decides to have a levonorgestrel IUS fitted. She needs support to continue with it as her menstrual loss is not immediately improved but after six months of use she is pleased to find that her periods are much more manageable.

Dysmenorrhoea and endometriosis

Case study 9.2

Miss Payne is referred to your gynaecology clinic with dysmenorrhoea at the age of 22 years. Over the last few months, her GP has prescribed simple analgesia which has become progressively less effective, although the patient is relieved that between her periods she has no significant discomfort. Although not in a relationship at present, she wishes to have children in the future, and she is concerned that her elder sister had recently had a total abdominal hysterectomy and bilateral salpingoophorectomy for endometriosis.

What issues you should cover

Although it is not possible to make a definitive diagnosis of endometriosis without visualising it, usually by laparoscopy for pelvic deposits or ultrasonography for endometriomas, the above history is highly suggestive. Nevertheless, it would be inappropriate to label the patient as having endometriosis without investigation. Consider alternative diagnoses such as idiopathic dysmenorrhoea, irritable bowel syndrome and PID. Ask her about her bowels and symptoms of infection. Vaginal examination may uncover significant tenderness if there are endometriotic deposits present or an enlarged ovary if it contains an endometrioma. If a woman is not trying to conceive and vaginal examination reveals no abnormality, symptomatic relief may be attempted using the combined oral contraceptive pill (monthly or tricycling by taking three packets sequentially without a break) with non-steroidal anti-inflammatory drugs during her periods.

However, if the pain is not controlled by simple treatment, or if the patient is anxious, then it would be appropriate to consider a laparoscopy to establish the diagnosis. Endometriosis may be controlled by progestogens, danazol or GnRH agonists (with add back oestrogen therapy if prolonged). Surgical treatment by ablation or excision laparoscopically or at laparotomy may prove necessary for control of the pain.[8] Further information on the investigation and management of endometriosis can be found on the RCOG website.[9]

Case study 9.2 continued

Miss Payne is extremely concerned at the possibility of endometriosis so you arrange a laparoscopy that reveals significant endometriosis and is treated with diathermy. Following this surgery the pain resolves, but the patient is counselled regarding the possibility of future recurrence.

Threatened miscarriage of pregnancy

Case study 9.3

The GP refers Mrs Loss to the early pregnancy assessment unit. She has had light vaginal bleeding but no pain at 8 weeks' gestation in her second pregnancy. However, in her first pregnancy she had miscarried at 7 weeks thus she is very concerned that she may miscarry again. She has read on the internet that progesterone may prevent miscarriages and she is desperate to do anything to save her pregnancy.

What issues you should cover

The description of early pregnancy loss as a miscarriage rather than an abortion is recommended. Although the terms have been used interchangeably, the term abortion is synonymous in the public's mind with therapeutic termination where a conscious decision to end the pregnancy, for whatever reason, has been made. Approximately 20% of clinically recognised pregnancies miscarry. At least half are due to chromosomal abnormalities in the fetus that are associated with increasing maternal age (but may affect women at any age). The psychological impact of miscarriage is significant and may affect the parents in the same way as any other bereavement. Ongoing support from primary care and increasingly from secondary care is an important aspect of management.

The main concern for this patient is whether the pregnancy is viable. Carry out an urgent pelvic ultrasound scan. This can also exclude the less likely, but very serious, possibility that she may have an ectopic pregnancy. Most parts of the UK can provide same-day access to an early pregnancy assessment unit that can provide emergency ultrasound scans and assist in patient management. The RCOG website provides more detailed guidance on the management of early pregnancy loss.[10]

Although it is very tempting to agree to patients' requests for treatments that may not cause harm, the current RCOG guidelines recommend that the value of progesterone to reduce the risk of even recurrent miscarriage remains unproven. At present progesterone should only be used in this condition in the context of research studies.

Recurrent miscarriage is defined as the loss of at least three pregnancies and affects 1 in 100 women. Couples may be distraught even after two miscarriages, particularly if associated with infertility and increased female age. Some treatments are controversial and even assessment of patients may differ between colleagues. This is a good topic for training while developing shared guidelines that are acceptable to all your colleagues in primary and secondary care. The RCOG guidelines *Investigation and Treatment of Couples with Recurrent Miscarriage* provide a good starting point for you to use.[11]

Case study 9.3 continued

Mrs Loss is delighted to see the fetal heart beating on the ultrasound scan. She wants to discuss whether she should stop her work as a secretary now to avoid any further risk to the pregnancy. You have read through the guidelines and are able to go through them with her. Although she has to decide for herself whether her anxiety merits stopping work, you advise her that normal activities are unlikely to make any difference to her risk of miscarriage.

Suspected ectopic pregnancy

Case study 9.4

The GP has referred Mrs Burst to the early pregnancy assessment unit complaining of severe lower abdominal pain. When you review her, the pain has settled a little after she has taken paracetamol. Her last period started two days earlier, but was 12 days late and was light even though she had an intrauterine contraceptive device *in situ*. However, her periods have always tended to be irregular so Mrs Burst thought nothing of this. Abdominal examination reveals lower abdominal tenderness and mild pyrexia.

What issues you should cover

Although the diagnosis is unclear, it is sensible to consider Mrs Burst has an ectopic pregnancy on the threshold of rupture until proven otherwise. Nevertheless, the possibility of other diagnoses including surgical pathology such as appendicitis must be considered. A sensitive pregnancy test may help resolve the diagnostic dilemma. If the pregnancy test is positive, then an early pregnancy problem is likely, whereas if the test is negative you may need to think further. Although abdominal examination can prove very useful, a transvaginal ultrasound examination can often establish a diagnosis. The differential diagnosis includes other gynaecological problems such as complications from ovarian cysts and acute pelvic inflammatory disease, for which the RCOG provides guidelines on management.[12]

In a woman with a suspected ectopic pregnancy measurement of HCG will help to determine:

- whether the patient is pregnant
- if the titres of HCG are consistent with a normal intrauterine pregnancy
- if the titres of HCG are low for the gestational age, suggestive of an abnormal pregnancy.

The threshold for detecting intrauterine pregnancy on transvaginal ultrasound ranges between 1000 and 1500 IU HCG. The detection of an adnexal mass or free fluid suggests an ectopic gestation although the woman's clinical condition and past history must be taken into account when deciding on her management. A combination of ultrasound assessment and maternal serum HCG levels help differentiate intrauterine from ectopic pregnancies and identify when a laparoscopy may be required. Quantitative determination of serum HCG may permit a conservative approach. The woman's symptoms are also important for deciding if and when to intervene. The majority of ectopic pregnancy can be managed laparoscopically. Salpingectomy is the most widely used treatment unless the contralateral tube is severely damaged when you should attempt to conserve the affected tube. Persistent trophoblastic disease occurs in up to 5% of salpingotomies and follow-up serum HCGs are essential.

Very early ectopic pregnancies may not be seen at laparoscopy, so monitor women until the serum HCG levels return to normal. Women who present with a ruptured ectopic pregnancy may not be suitable for a laparoscopic approach and laparotomy may be necessary.

Case study 9.4 continued

Mrs Burst is found to have a high serum HCG level with no sign of an intrauterine pregnancy and free fluid in the pelvis. In view of the high index of suspicion of a ruptured ectopic pregnancy, a laparoscopy is performed revealing a ruptured right tubal ectopic pregnancy so you perform a laparoscopic salpingectomy.

Primary amenorrhoea

Primary amenorrhoea is defined as the failure to establish menstruation by the age of 14 years if there are no signs of secondary sexual maturation, or by the age of 16 years if normal secondary sexual characteristics are developing.[13] In hospital practice you may encounter a range of complex underlying conditions including intersex, congenital anomalies and endocrine dysfunctions, but many cases are managed in primary care with comprehensive guidance on the management of amenorrhoea in the community available from Prodigy.[14]

Case study 9.5

Miss Little attends with her mother who does all the talking. Her mother says she is worried as her daughter, who has just had her 15th birthday, has not yet had a period.

What issues you should cover

If this information is not volunteered you may need to ask specifically about the following points.

- Establish with Miss Little that her mother does mean that she has never had a period, not just none for two months! It is possible, too, for ovulation to occur prior to a first period. Always think about pregnancy.
- Find out the age when the mother and any sisters started their periods, as it may be constitutional. That is, the pulsatile production of GnRH occurs later in some families.
- Determine if there is any family history of any genetic disorders such as Turner's syndrome (if it is mild with only short stature and web neck it may escape notice until puberty).
- Chronic illness, weight loss, anorexia, high levels of exercise or stress can cause hypothalamic dysfunction. Breast milk production might suggest prolactin excess.
- Cyclical abdominal pain may suggest a genitourinary abnormality such as an imperforate hymen or an absent vagina with a functioning uterus.
- Enquire if there has been previous treatment e.g. with chemotherapy, as you may not know about previous treatment for a brain tumour, or for a hydrocephalus.

The examination

Check her weight and height to establish her body mass index (BMI). If the BMI is less than 19, regular menstruation is unlikely. Ask Miss Little if she would like a chaperone for any examination. She may prefer to have a nurse present, rather than her mother, and this gives you another opportunity to check the history (e.g. about risk of pregnancy or anorexia) from her. Chart the second-ary sexual characteristics (*see* Table 9.1). Look for signs of hypothyroidism, hirsutes, and features of Turner's syndrome that would indicate specific investigations. If she consents to you looking at her external genitalia, record your findings, but pelvic examination is not useful or appropriate at this stage. If she has secondary sexual characteristics and you are at all suspicious, do a pregnancy test.

Table 9.1: Tanner's stages of puberty in females[15]

Stage	Breast	Pubic hair
1: Pre-adolescent	Only papillae are elevated.	Vellus hair only and hair is similar to development over anterior abdominal wall (i.e. no pubic hair).
2	Breast bud and papilla are elevated and a small mount is present; areola diameter is enlarged.	There is sparse growth of long, slightly pigmented, downy hair or only slightly curled hair, appearing along labia.
3	Further enlargement of breast mound; increased palpable glandular tissue.	Hair is darker, coarser, more curled, and spreads to the pubic junction.
4	Areola and papilla are elevated to form a second mound above the level of the rest of the breast.	Adult-type hair; area covered is less than that in most adults; there is no spread to the medial surface of thighs.
5: Adult	Adult mature breast; recession of areola to the mound of breast tissue, rounding of the breast mound, and projection of only the papillae are evident.	Adult-type hair with increased spread to medial surface of thighs; distribution is as an inverse triangle.

Case study 9.5 continued

Miss Little has some secondary sexual characteristics equivalent, you think, to stage 3. Both she and her mother are small and thin and her BMI is only 19. You discuss with her about avoiding smoking and having a good diet. You advise her to increase her calcium intake, how to ensure that she has sufficient sunlight for vitamin D production and to take plenty of weight-bearing exercise to maximise her bone mass. You arrange to see her again in six months if she has not started her periods, or before then if any new symptoms appear.

Secondary amenorrhoea and oligomenorrhoea

Case study 9.6

Mrs Reed, a miserable-looking thin woman of 39 years, normally attends another doctor quite frequently with multiple somatic complaints, so you are a little wary. She tells you that the practice nurse suggested that she consulted you as she has not had a proper period for months and is feeling terrible. On enquiry, you eventually determine that her last episode of bleeding was about eight or nine weeks ago and she complained to her usual doctor about how heavy it was at the time, but she has not had a regular cycle for years.

What issues you should cover

Exclude pregnancy with a pregnancy test. It may seem obvious, but check that she is not receiving a progestogen-only method of contraception (*see* Chapter 5), that would give her irregular periods.

You would usually wait until six months of amenorrhoea until putting in train other investigations, but you might have a lower threshold for investigations in this chronically unwell woman.

As in primary amenorrhoea, chronic illness or stress can cause hypothalamic dysfunction. She may have problems arising from weight loss or anorexia or possibly high levels of exercise, in which case you should enquire regarding visual disturbance. Breast milk production might suggest prolactin excess. Avoid examining the breasts for expression of milk if you are going to take blood for a prolactin level as it may raise the level. Ask about symptoms suggestive of thyroid disease. Check that she is not taking any antipsychotic or other medication that might affect hypothalamic function. Look out for symptoms or signs that would suggest PCOS which occurs in 30% of women with secondary amenorrhoea.[16] Not all patients with PCOS have obesity with hyperpigmentation of the skin folds, but she might have excess body hair, alopecia, acne and a history of difficulty with conception. She might have similar symptoms and signs with rarer conditions like Cushing's syndrome or, if excess body hair has developed rapidly, adrenal hyperplasia, an adrenal tumour or an ovarian androgen-producing tumour.

Symptoms of hot flushes might suggest premature ovarian failure (*see* Chapter 10) and may be associated with autoimmune conditions such as hypothyroidism, diabetes or Addison's disease. Occasionally structural abnormalities of the vagina, stenosis of the cervix or adhesions in the uterus can cause amenorrhoea, usually with complaints of abdominal pain.

Choosing your investigations

Always do a pregnancy test. Take blood for the levels of FSH, LH, prolactin (*see* Table 9.2 for interpretation in common conditions) and thyroid function in all patients with secondary amenorrhoea. Testosterone levels may be useful in patients with hirsutes. If the levels of testosterone are in the male range, an adrenal or androgenic tumour may be present prompting specialist referral.

Oestradiol blood levels vary too much to be useful, but a progestogen challenge test can show that adequate oestrogens are present. Do not use this test if you suspect any structural obstruction to the menstrual flow. If you give medroxyprogesterone acetate 10 mg once a day for 7 days, a withdrawal bleed will follow unless oestradiol levels are low.

Pelvic ultrasound may show the classic picture of polycystic ovaries with their string of pearls appearance from the multiple small peripherally situated cysts.

Table 9.2: Hormone results in common causes of amenorrhoea

	FSH	*LH*	*Prolactin*	*Testosterone*
Hyperprolactinaemia (requires further investigation regarding cause)	Normal or low	Normal or low	High	Normal
Polycystic ovarian syndrome	Normal	Normal or slightly raised	Normal or moderate rise	Slightly raised
Premature menopause	Very high	High	Normal	Normal
Hypothalamic e.g. with weight loss, excess exercise, stress	Normal or low	Normal or low	Normal	Normal

If you are still uncertain about the underlying cause, or about how to manage a condition you have identified, you might wish to refer to a gynaecologist. A patient with a high prolactin will require computerised tomography or magnetic resonance imaging and specialist advice from an endocrinologist.

Correction of underlying causes such as anorexia may require referral to a psychologist or psychiatrist, but lesser degrees of weight loss or over-exercising can be managed in the community.

PCOS responds best to weight loss. Patients often require treatment for associated lipid disorders, diabetes or hypertension. Treatment with metformin may be considered but evidence for prevention of long-term adverse outcomes is not yet available. You could consult the management guidance.[17]

Case study 9.6 continued

Mrs Reed's investigations are all normal except for a slightly raised prolactin level. You tell her that her tests do not suggest that she is menopausal as she assumed. You suggest that she keeps a record of her menstrual loss over the next six months. Later in the year, you hear from her regular doctor that she has moved onto other complaints and has not mentioned her periods again!

Collecting data to demonstrate your learning, competence, performance and standards of service delivery

Example cycle of evidence 9.1

- Focus: clinical care
- Other relevant focus: maintaining good medical practice

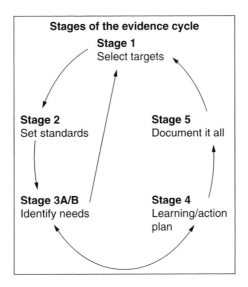

Stages of the evidence cycle

Stage 1
Select targets

Stage 2
Set standards

Stage 3A/B
Identify needs

Stage 4
Learning/action plan

Stage 5
Document it all

> **Case study 9.7**
>
> Mrs Razor is referred to your gynaecology clinic troubled that her periods have become irregular. She is unhappy with her body image and she wishes to lose weight, which has been gradually increasing since her 40th birthday last year. She now weighs 90 kg at a height of 1.65 metres. As you discuss her problems, it becomes apparent that there is something that is causing her worry and embarrassment. Eventually she summons the courage to tell you that her main problem is that she has more frequently needed to shave her legs, and she is worried that she is becoming more 'hairy'.

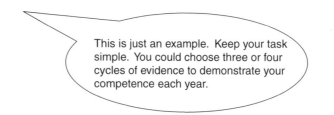

This is just an example. Keep your task simple. You could choose three or four cycles of evidence to demonstrate your competence each year.

Stage 1: Select your aspirations for good practice

The excellent doctor:

- is sympathetic to the concerns of patients and recognises the presenting complaint may not always be the main concern
- provides patients with the opportunity and the confidence to discuss sensitive issues.

Stage 2: Set the standards for your outcomes

Outcomes might include:

- the way learning is applied
- a learnt skill
- a protocol
- a strategy that is implemented
- meeting recommended standards.

- Demonstrate consistent best practice in management of PCOS and related problems.
- Show enthusiasm when patients consult with obesity.

Stage 3A: Identify your learning needs

- Self-assess and reflect on your own learning needs in respect of PCOS with regard to diagnosis and management.
- Conduct a significant event audit of delayed diagnosis in a case of PCOS.

Stage 3B: Identify your service needs

> Any of the needs assessment exercises in 3A may also reveal service needs.

- Review the advice provided to obese individuals who wish to lose weight – how does it compare against national guidelines?
- Audit the records of patients with important comorbidities such as diabetes mellitus and hypertension to see if appropriate advice about diet and their weight has been given to these patients.

Stage 4: Make and carry out a learning and action plan

- The RCOG provides guidelines on the long-term consequences of PCOS, which may provide a useful update on this condition.[17]
- As there are many controversial aspects regarding PCOS you may find it useful to discuss this condition with a local specialist or attend a lecture on the subject where you can discuss your queries.
- Arrange a presentation in your hospital or practice either by yourself or from an invited speaker to discuss the implications and management of obesity and PCOS.

Stage 5: Document your learning, competence, performance and standards of service delivery

- Write your own notes about the recognition and management of PCOS and keep a record of key references including useful website pages in your learning portfolio.
- For later reference make a note of the development webpage for NICE guidelines on *Obesity: the prevention, identification, evaluation, treatment and weight maintenance of overweight and obesity in adults.*[18]

Case study 9.7 continued

Following confirmation of the diagnosis of PCOS by ultrasound scan and slight elevation of serum androgens, Mrs Razor is relieved to hear your explanation of her symptoms. Recognising the importance of weight reduction, Mrs Razor has altered her lifestyle to increase the amount of exercise and is now on a long-term diet plan aiming for gradual but sustained weight reduction.

Example cycle of evidence 9.2

- Focus: relationships with patients

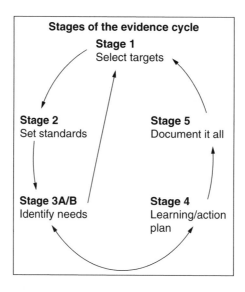

Stages of the evidence cycle

Stage 1
Select targets

Stage 2
Set standards

Stage 5
Document it all

Stage 3A/B
Identify needs

Stage 4
Learning/action plan

Case study 9.8

Mrs Weeds is a 63-year-old widow, who is urgently referred to the gynaecology outpatient clinic as she reported to her GP that she has started to bleed vaginally.

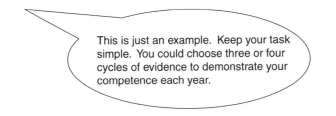

This is just an example. Keep your task simple. You could choose three or four cycles of evidence to demonstrate your competence each year.

Stage 1: Select your aspirations for good practice

The excellent doctor:

- will support patients at time of particular stress such as around the time of possible detection of cancer
- will be aware when a minor symptom may indicate the possibility of a serious condition and convey this information to patients.

Stage 2: Set the standards for your outcomes

Outcomes might include:

- the way learning is applied
- a learnt skill
- a protocol
- a strategy that is implemented
- meeting recommended standards.

- Ensure appropriate patient education and screening processes are in place to detect gynaecological cancers at an early stage.

Stage 3A: Identify your learning needs

- Consider what you know and what patients should know about endometrial cancer, cervical cancer, ovarian cancer and vulval cancer.
- Compare your initial diagnoses with the final outcome in the last 20 patients that you reviewed with postmenopausal bleeding. Did you identify the patients most at risk of cancer and minimise the distress to patients who had a low risk of cancer?
- Self-assess if you are able to inform patients of the significance of the symptoms and signs to look out for uterine cancer without causing alarm. Invite retrospective feedback from patients.

Stage 3B: Identify your service needs

> Any of the needs assessment exercises in 3A may also reveal service needs.

- Review the quantity and quality of patient information sources e.g. leaflets and websites for gynaecological cancer and self-assess your and colleagues' knowledge and skills.
- Consider whether a one-stop clinic for postmenopausal bleeding may be possible in your hospital, or if you have such a service, check that it is run optimally.

Stage 4: Make and carry out a learning and action plan

- Ensure that you are aware of current best practice in screening and initial management of gynaecological cancers by reading, discussion with colleagues and attending an update lecture or workshop.
- Visit another hospital that runs a one-stop clinic for vaginal bleeding and compare this with your practice to see if yours may be improved.

Stage 5: Document your learning, competence, performance and standards of service delivery

- Although verbal praise (as below) is very satisfying, a written statement could form valuable evidence for your portfolio. You could ask the patient to drop you a line after viewing the website material so that you could know whether to recommend this site to other patients and to provide you with a written record of the patient's views.
- Keep a record of the activities you undertake from above and file this in your learning portfolio.

Case study 9.8 continued

Two weeks later Mrs Weeds returns to the gynaecology clinic with her daughter. She has had an ultrasound scan and outpatient hysteroscopy, which confirmed a diagnosis of endometrial cancer. She has seen the hospital consultant who had explained what this meant and arranged for her to be admitted shortly for a hysterectomy. The consultant has asked you to complete a pre-operative clerking, during which her daughter enquired if there was any website they could access for information to read at their own pace. The patient was pleased with your sympathetic management when she initially presented and is delighted that you are able to point them to the CancerBACUP website.[19]

Example cycle of evidence 9.3

- Focus: working with colleagues
- Other relevant focus: teaching and training

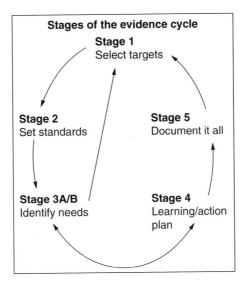

Stages of the evidence cycle

Stage 1
Select targets

Stage 2
Set standards

Stage 5
Document it all

Stage 3A/B
Identify needs

Stage 4
Learning/action plan

Case study 9.9
You are a PwSI in women's health, leading on infertility management for your team and with the help of the local hospital infertility consultant are drafting guidelines for the practice for recurrent miscarriage.

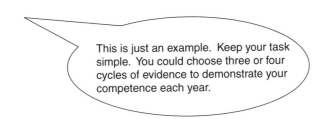

This is just an example. Keep your task simple. You could choose three or four cycles of evidence to demonstrate your competence each year.

Stage 1: Select your aspirations for good practice

The excellent doctor:

- respects the views of colleagues and patients when developing group guidelines on best practice
- helps to train professional colleagues and share knowledge.

Stage 2: Set the standards for your outcomes

Outcomes might include:

- the way learning is applied
- a learnt skill
- a protocol
- a strategy that is implemented
- meeting recommended standards.

- Develop practice guidelines for management of recurrent miscarriage considering the availability of local resources and local opinion and best practice from national guidelines.[11]

Stage 3A: Identify your learning needs

- Review your knowledge of recurrent miscarriage tests against the above national guidelines, checking the local costs of these investigations and any other routine tests performed locally.
- Review the significance and interpretation of the tests, such as for thrombophilia and antiphospholipid screening, from the evidence presented in the national guidelines.

Stage 3B: Identify your service needs

Any of the needs assessment exercises in 3A may also reveal service needs.

- Assess current practice by auditing the investigations performed of the last 10 patients presenting with recurrent miscarriage.
- Compare the management of recurrent miscarriage with the standard management for miscarriage through a questionnaire of patients' experiences.
- Also consider that reference to the guidelines on the management of less common forms of miscarriage such as hydatidiform mole may be usefully mentioned as a special circumstance for awareness of your colleagues.[20]

Stage 4: Make and carry out a learning and action plan

- Arrange a visit to your practice from a local specialist preferably from the local recurrent miscarriage clinic if you have one. Invite others from across your PCO to join in to discuss local guidelines.
- Discuss management with colleagues and draft, then agree, consensus guidelines.
- Produce a tutorial for your colleagues on hydatidiform mole.

Stage 5: Document your learning, competence, performance and standards of service delivery

- Document brief minutes of meetings to produce guidelines, for inclusion in your portfolio with a copy of the final guidelines.
- Record the audit of the investigations performed of the last 10 patients presenting with recurrent miscarriage and the patient questionnaires.
- File a copy of the tutorial on hydatidiform mole.

Case study 9.9 continued

You find that drafting guidelines for your practice or the local area is a good educational process that encourages you in working effectively with your colleagues.

References

1 www.rcog.org.uk/guidelines.asp?PageID=108&GuidelineID=28

2 Vessey M, Villard L, Mackintosh M *et al.* (1992) The epidemiology of hysterectomy: findings in a large cohort study. *British Journal of Obstetrics and Gynaecology.* **99**: 402–7.

3 Porteous A and Prentice A (2003) Medical management of dysfunctional uterine bleeding. *Reviews in Gynaecological Practice.* **3**: 81–4.

4 Lethaby A, Cooke I and Rees M (2002) Progesterone/progestogen releasing intrauterine system for heavy menstrual bleeding (Cochrane Review). In: *The Cochrane Library, Issue 4, 2002.* Update Software, Oxford.

5 Barrington JW and Bowen-Simpkins P (1997) The levonorgestrel intrauterine system in the management of menorrhagia. *British Journal of Obstetrics and Gynaecology.* **104**: 614–16.

6 Sowter MC (2003) New surgical treatments for menorrhagia. *Lancet.* **361**: 1456–8.

7 Pron G, Bennett J, Common A *et al.* and Ontario Uterine Fibroid Embolization Collaborative Group (2003) The Ontario Uterine Fibroid Embolization Trial. Part 2. Uterine fibroid reduction and symptom relief after uterine artery embolization for fibroids. *Fertility and Sterility.* **79:** 120–7.

8 Winkel CA (2003) Evaluation and management of women with endometriosis. *Obstetrics and Gynecology.* **102:** 397–408.

9 www.rcog.org.uk/guidelines.asp?PageID=106&GuidelineID=10

10 www.rcog.org.uk/guidelines.asp?PageID=106&GuidelineID=8

11 www.rcog.org.uk/guidelines.asp?PageID=106&GuidelineID=46

12 www.rcog.org.uk/guidelines.asp?PageID=106&GuidelineID=49

13 Edmonds DK (ed.) (1999) *Dewhurst's Textbook of Obstetrics and Gynaecology For Postgraduates* (6e). Blackwell Science, Oxford.

14 www.prodigy.nhs.uk/guidance.asp?gt=Amenorrhoea

15 Marshall WA and Tanner JM (1969) Variations in pattern of pubertal changes in girls. *Archives of Disease in Childhood.* **44:** 291–303.

16 Hopkinson ZE, Sattar N, Fleming R *et al.* (1998) Polycystic ovarian syndrome: the metabolic syndrome comes to gynaecology. *British Medical Journal.* **317:** 329–32.

17 www.rcog.org.uk/guidelines.asp?PageID=106&GuidelineID=50

18 www.nice.org.uk

19 www.cancerbacup.org.uk/info/womb.htm

20 www.rcog.org.uk/guidelines.asp?PageID=106&GuidelineID=21

10

The menopause

Managing the menopause encompasses far more than just knowing about hormone replacement therapy (HRT). However, the plethora of articles recently published and hitting the headlines have made women and their doctors much more aware of the indications, risks and benefits of HRT. If you are to be competent in advising patients you need to be able to dispel the myths and give advice from an evidence-based viewpoint as far as possible – and acknowledge that there is still much to be discovered. Bear in mind that much of the evidence published recently has been from studies carried out on women older than the usual age for consulting about menopausal symptoms, or on selected populations, and the conclusions may not be relevant to the individual referred to you. This chapter provides a broad overview and the British Menopause Society in collaboration with the RCOG has developed a special interest training programme covering the menopause (*see* Box 10.1).

Box 10.1: Requirements of the British Menopause Society and Royal College of Obstetricians and Gynaecologists for menopause special skills training[1]

Entry criteria

1   Passed Part 2 MRCOG or hold an equivalent qualification
2   Satisfactorily completed the core logbook requirements
3   Obtained a satisfactory Year 3 RITA

Training programme components

1   Training under the supervision of an identified preceptor for one year
2   Attend a theoretical course that should provide the essential knowledge component of training for this module supplemented by personal study
3   Attend at least 30 menopause or related clinics (including bone densitometry clinics, dual energy X-ray absorptiometry (DEXA), cardiology clinics and breast clinics)
4   Complete 10 referenced case reports and a clinical audit on a subject related to the menopause
5   Satisfactory completion of logbook defining the skills required for the management of the menopause

---

> **Case study 10.1**
>
> You are asked by your consultant to staff the menopause clinic. An experienced hospital practitioner usually runs this clinic with a specialist nurse but the doctor is on sick leave. Mrs Teacher, a 46-year-old woman, is referred to the clinic with irregular periods. She says that she thinks she is 'on the change' and is worried as she remembers her mother having lots of problems. She says that she has to be on top form all the time in her job. She says that she has doubts about HRT and wants to know what else she might take.

What issues you should cover

Age

Usually the menopause happens between the ages of 48 and 54 years, but it may occur outside these ages. The median age of menopause is 51 years. The *menopause* is the permanent stopping of menstruation resulting from loss of ovarian follicle activity. The natural menopause is defined as being after 12 months of no menstruation, so can only be decided after the event.

The *perimenopause* includes the time beginning with the first features of the approaching menopause, such as hot flushes or menstrual irregularity. It ends 12 months after the last menstrual period. The perimenopause occurs over a very varied time interval and can sometimes last several years with menopausal symptoms, and menstrual periods, coming and going. The *postmenopause* starts with the last menstrual period but cannot be dated with certainty until 12 months have occurred without menstruation.

A *premature menopause* is usually defined as the permanent cessation of menstrual periods due to loss of ovarian follicular activity occurring before 40 years of age. A *surgical menopause* occurs when the ovaries are removed. This is sometimes done together with a hysterectomy and causes a sudden drop in female hormone level, often with severe symptoms.

Timing of her last period

Mrs Teacher could be having menopausal symptoms even if she is still having menstrual periods (perimenopause) but you would also want to think about alternative reasons for hot sweats (e.g. anxiety, pyrexia) or psychological symptoms (e.g. worsening premenstrual syndrome or depression).[2]

If she has not had a recent period, ensure that she is not pregnant. Many women think that they cannot become pregnant if they are coming up to 50 years of age and stop using contraception. If she is at risk of pregnancy, arrange a pregnancy test and discuss contraceptive precautions with her.[3,4]

If she has been having periods, she may be worried because she has missed periods or had them more frequently and that the amount of loss is different. Periods may become closer together because the luteal phase is shortened when ovulation is not occurring. You will recall that the luteal phase occurs after ovulation when the corpus luteum, formed from the cells around the released ovum, produces progesterone to maintain the endometrium ready for a fertilised ovum. Irregular loss of the endometrium occurs when insufficient progesterone is produced. This loss is light or absent if oestrogen levels are also lowered. The loss can be heavy if oestrogen levels are fluctuating and sometimes high enough to increase the thickness of the endometrium.

Irregular vaginal loss

You will need to know more about her irregular periods. If they are heavy irregular periods that are more frequent, or if she has intermenstrual bleeding, ensure that the cause is hormonal fluctuations and not endometrial hyperplasia or carcinoma, before discussing management of her perimenopausal state. You might want to obtain an endometrial sample to check for hyperplasia or measure the endometrial thickness with vaginal ultrasound.

Hot flushes

If Mrs Teacher has been having hot flushes establish how often they are occurring, how much of a nuisance they are and whether they are disturbing her sleep. Being woken several times a night can lead to irritability and loss of concentration the following day, especially if she has to get out of bed to change nightwear or sheets because of sweating.

Vaginal dryness

Thinning of the vaginal walls, less lubrication and discomfort with sexual intercourse tend to occur after several years of lowered hormone levels, but some women will develop this earlier. Use direct questions as many women will not volunteer this information but will be grateful for a chance to discuss it.

Formication

You may also need to ask about this condition of feeling as if something is crawling just under the skin, as many women do not like to mention it. They often think that it is a sign of a psychiatric illness and are very reassured to discover that it can occur as a symptom of the menopause.

Bladder symptoms

Urgency and frequency of micturition are often associated with vaginal dryness and she may have noticed a tendency to have more frequent urinary tract infections. Incontinence or difficulties passing urine are more likely to be associated with structural abnormalities such as urogenital prolapse.

Psychological symptoms

Contrary to popular belief, there is no clear evidence that changes in hormone levels at the menopause can cause depression. Most women do not have major mood changes around their menopause and those that do usually have other reasons for their symptoms.[5,6] The physical changes of the menopause may make it more difficult to cope with the many major life stresses that occur in 40–60 year olds of both sexes. If psychological symptoms are prominent, enquire about other stressful events such as:

- parents ageing and becoming dependent
- deaths of family or friends
- loss of a partner through death, separation or divorce
- children leaving home
- demanding workload
- family worries such as partner's job, children's marriages, etc
- poor health
- money worries
- coming to terms with her own ageing.

Worries about osteoporosis[7,8]

If Mrs Teacher is concerned about having thinning of her bones, establish if this is because she has symptoms of aching or swelling of her joints. Symptoms will need independent evaluation for their cause but they are often part of the ageing process rather than being due to menopausal changes.

A family history such as a mother or sister with osteoporosis is associated with a higher risk of developing it herself. Other factors that might give her a higher risk are:

- an established menopause before the age of 45 years
- being underweight
- smoking
- taking little physical exercise
- treatment with corticosteroids
- a poor diet with little calcium or vitamin D intake
- excess alcohol intake
- a fragility fracture (one occurring with minimal trauma such as slipping over)
- having a medical condition such as:
  - rheumatoid arthritis
  - malabsorption syndromes (Crohn's disease, ulcerative colitis, gluten sensitivity)
  - liver disease
  - parathyroid disease
  - hyperthyroidism or excess replacement therapy for hypothyroidism.

Reasons for a hormonal blood test

Many women ask if they can have a blood test to determine whether they are 'on the change'. If a woman has already stopped having periods, there is little point unless she requires investigation because she might have a premature menopause. The variable level of hormones in people having periods makes hormonal blood tests largely irrelevant too (*see* Box 10.2). The only indication for blood tests is if the history is suggestive of a condition other than a straightforward menopausal transition.

Box 10.2: Blood tests for menopausal symptoms

Follicle stimulating hormone (FSH) is only helpful if the level is in the menopausal range (over 30 IU/l). The level fluctuates widely when a woman is still having menstrual loss and is going through the perimenopause. The level is controlled by the pulsatile release of GnRH from the hypothalamus, and is affected by feedback from oestrogen and progesterone levels as well as by inhibin. Several measurements over a period of time may be required if a premature menopause is suspected.

Oestradiol levels are not useful in the diagnosis of the menopause, either premature or at the usual time, because of the variation in levels from day to day and even at various times of day. Oestradiol levels can be used to check the levels of circulating hormone before replacement of subcutaneous implants of oestrogen, or to check levels absorbed from the skin or mucous membranes. Oestrogen given orally is mainly converted to oestrone so that oestradiol levels are not helpful.

Thyroid function tests may be useful when doubt arises as to whether symptoms are actually menopausal. Tiredness, weight gain, hair loss and flushes may indicate an underactive thyroid rather than ovarian failure.

What she may know about the menopause

This first consultation might focus on patient education including what Mrs Teacher can do herself to combat the effects of the menopause.[8] She may want to discuss:

- identifying the things that trigger the flushes, e.g. hot drinks, caffeine, spicy food, alcohol, and reducing or avoiding them
- wearing layers of clothing so that some can be removed easily when she has a flush
- relaxation techniques to avoid feeling stressed and rushed, as anxiety can make flushes more frequent
- taking regular exercise, eating healthily and avoiding smoking[9]
- using lubricants to make sexual intercourse more comfortable
- using plant substances that have similar effects to those of oestrogens.[10] There is some evidence that phytoestrogens might be helpful. The two important groups of foods containing phytoestrogens are: isoflavones that are found in soybeans, chick peas, red clover and probably other legumes; and lignans that are found in linseeds and smaller amounts in cereal bran, vegetables, legumes and fruit. However, phytoestrogens are unlikely to have a major effect on symptoms[11]
- using other alternative therapies, e.g. acupuncture or homeopathy although little firm evidence exists that they are helpful.[12,13]

Be cautious about the claims for other herbal treatments, some of which may interact with prescribed medications (e.g. warfarin, antidepressants). Others may contain toxic chemicals such as pesticides, mercury, arsenic and lead. Black cohosh has been approved in Germany for treatment of the menopause, and St John's Wort can help with mild depressive symptoms.

Progesterone cream is sold for treatment of menopausal symptoms. Insufficient is absorbed to be bone-protective, or to provide protection for the endometrium if oestrogen replacement therapy is used, but some women report lessening of symptom severity.

Advising on hormone replacement therapy (HRT)

If you have had a long consultation already, you might at this stage give Mrs Teacher some information on HRT to take away with her. You might want to check that the information available in the clinic is up to date because of the rapidly changing advice due to recent publications. Establishing a small patient library with books and websites, videos and leaflets relating to the menopause will be helpful and informative for patients, but you may need to supplement or modify this with the most recently published information.[14,15] She can return to see you better informed and better able to discuss the advantages and disadvantages of treatment.

Continuing management

Case study 10.2

Ms Mind is your next patient in the clinic. She is 51 years old and has been referred by her GP, who wants your opinion about whether she should continue on HRT and if so, what type. She is a tall, thin woman who smells of cigarettes. She tells you that she used to be a psychiatric nurse but is now in private practice as a therapist. She says that she thinks that her GP wants her to stop HRT, but she wants to continue. She has been on several different sequential preparations over the last four years, changing because of irregular bleeding or symptoms of the premenstrual syndrome during the progestogen phase. She implies that her GP knows little about the problems women have. She is relatively happy on the preparation she is on at present (that contains dydrogesterone as the progestogen) but wants to avoid having any periods. She tells you that a friend of hers has an implant every six months and she understands that she could have this done at the clinic.

The consensus opinion in the UK is that HRT should be used for symptom relief, at the lowest dose and for the shortest time compatible with the control of unacceptable symptoms.[16–19] Find out the consensus of opinion among the colleagues with whom you work. Many health professionals are poorly informed about the risks and benefits of HRT and may have biased opinions based on incomplete or inaccurate information. You need to be able to discuss the options from evidence-based information. Some conditions that have received publicity recently may need specific discussion and you should be aware of the conclusions from the studies and their limitations. HRT should not be recommended when there is an increased risk of the following conditions, or for the prevention of these conditions:[17–19]

- *cardiovascular disease*: the risk of heart attacks and strokes is slightly increased, mainly in the first couple of years of use
- *venous thromboembolism*: there is a 2–3-fold increase in risk with oral preparations. This may not apply to transdermal therapy. The background risk of thrombosis in menopausal women is about 1 in 10 000 women per year. Using HRT will increase this by about two to four extra women in every 10 000 developing a thrombosis each year
- *endometrial cancer*: oestrogen-only and sequential combined HRT appear to increase the risk slightly, but continuous combined therapy appears to be slightly protective
- *breast cancer*: the excess risk of breast cancer appears to be similar to that attributable to a late menopause. Although small in absolute terms, it has provoked much alarm. Combined therapy was found in recent studies to give the greatest risk (an additional six per thousand cases after five years of use), oestrogen-only therapy giving only a very small extra risk (an additional 1.5 per thousand cases after five years of use), and tibolone (*see* Box 10.4) an intermediate risk. In women aged 50–64 years, the baseline risk is 32 per 1000, so this increases the risk to 33.5 per 1000 for those taking oestrogen-only therapy and 38 per 1000 for combined therapy users. Five years after stopping HRT, the woman's risk of breast cancer is the same as for women who have never taken it. If women are taking HRT at the time their breast cancer is diagnosed, their life expectancy does not seem to be reduced. It is not known if this is because cancers are diagnosed at an earlier stage in HRT users or because the HRT has an effect on the cancer.[18–22]

The previous suggestion that HRT might protect against Alzheimer's disease has not been confirmed, although the greater risk of dementia shown in older women might be due to the prothrombotic effects of HRT.

HRT is protective against osteoporosis and prevents fractures. However, other therapies, such as biphosphonates, should be considered if there are no other indications for HRT, if lifestyle changes and calcium and vitamin D supplements are insufficient.

Most other conditions appear to be unaffected by HRT although colorectal cancer incidence appears to be reduced.

Take a history for conditions that might be affected by HRT. Physical examination should include measurement of her blood pressure and BMI. Clinical breast examination may give false reassurance but you might encourage breast awareness so that she would spot any early changes in appearance. Mammography has a higher sensitivity and specificity for breast cancer than clinical examination. Participation in national screening programmes should be encouraged. You should be familiar with local arrangements for mammography so that you can discuss when invitations are likely to arrive, and explain what is involved. Women should also be encouraged to participate in the cervical screening programme.

Establish with Ms Mind what expectations she has of the HRT. If she still has some menopausal symptoms, such as hot flushes, or has had a return of symptoms in any intervals when HRT has been stopped, she may well be keen to continue. She may have misplaced beliefs that ageing will be delayed or mental agility preserved.

Explain that HRT consists of an oestrogen, which is usually combined with a progestogen in women who have not had a hysterectomy. She could take the hormone(s) by different routes: oral, transdermal, subcutaneous, intranasal and vaginal. Most women will now be started on 1 mg oestradiol orally, 50 µg transdermally, or 25 mg implanted oestradiol, unless the woman has a premature menopause or also has severe osteoporosis.

Women may be given an oestrogen subcutaneous implant after a total hysterectomy and bilateral oophorectomy but this method of administration can be difficult to manage (*see* Box 10.3). In some clinics, testosterone is added to the implant procedure for relief of complaints of lack of sexual drive. As Ms Mind has not had a hysterectomy, she would still need to have endometrial protection from a progestogen. Discuss with her why she liked this idea. If her friend has received testosterone together with the oestrogen implant, she may believe that this type of HRT would improve her sex life.

Box 10.3:   Management of oestrogen implants

Use of subcutaneous implants was associated with tachyphylaxis i.e. menopausal symptoms returned and a further implant was given even while the blood levels of oestradiol were high. Very high levels of oestradiol could be attained after repeated implants. Although the risk of this occurring appeared low, some women were intolerant of symptoms and demanded early replacement of the implant. The management now advised is not to replace an implant until oestradiol levels are no higher than 400 pmol/l.[23] The implant is usually replaced at intervals of 4–8 months and can be inserted subcutaneously into the abdominal wall by anyone trained in the technique who is able to monitor the oestrogen level before replacement.

If Ms Mind was interested in a hormone replacement to help with her sexual life, she might want to discuss tibolone. Tibolone is a synthetic hormone that has mixed oestrogenic, progestogenic and androgenic actions, and is used by women who do not want to have bleeding (*see* Box 10.4).

Box 10.4:   How tibolone differs from oestrogen plus progestogen replacement therapy[24]

- It alleviates menopausal symptoms like oestrogen, but its effect on the endometrium is like that of progestogen. Cyclical bleeding is not promoted.
- Vaginal cell maturation is normalised and symptomatic atrophic vaginitis is relieved with reduction in vaginal dryness and dyspareunia.
- Randomised studies have shown improvements in mood compared with placebo and similar effects on adverse mood to conventional HRT.
- It significantly reduces SHBG and has some androgenic effects. Improvements in sexual functioning are greater than those seen with conventional HRT.
- It has oestrogenic effects on bone density.
- Tibolone inhibits proliferation of human breast cells. The incidence of breast tenderness is low and breast density is not increased unlike with conventional HRT. It is not known if this translates into clinical significance for the risk of breast cancer, but the Million Women study found an incidence of breast cancer higher than that for oestrogen, but lower than for combined hormonal HRT.[21]
- The literature does not report any increase in thrombotic events in women taking tibolone (but this may be due to the small numbers of women taking it).

Tibolone does not suit every woman and may provide inadequate relief of symptoms in some women. Some complain of progestogen-like side-effects.

Selecting HRT

If menstruation has not stopped, a GP or specialist is likely to have started HRT with a monthly (or three-monthly) sequential cyclical preparation to try to promote a regular bleeding pattern. Once no menstruation has occurred for 12 months, a continuous combined, no bleed, preparation can be tried. It is sensible to become familiar with a few of the large range of HRT therapies available rather than attempting to know about all the preparations in detail. You will probably need to establish which preparations are in common use in the clinic in which you are working and why. It can help you to draw up a list of therapies that patients are most likely to ask about, and you should be able to give the rationale for prescribing in a particular manner. The cost of the preparation must feature in the decision-making process of what to prescribe, but equally important is determining the acceptability to the woman. Oral medication is generally cheaper than other options, but the woman should have an opportunity to discuss exactly what she would prefer. If you build up a supply of placebo options that patients can handle, it will help women to decide which type they would prefer to use.

Protecting the endometrium in women who have not had a hysterectomy

Progestogens are added to reduce the risk of hyperplasia and carcinoma of the endometrium that occurs with unopposed oestrogen. Women who have had endometrial ablation need progestogens, as it cannot be assumed that all the endometrium has been removed. Standard sequential or continuous combined therapy contain suitable levels of progestogen to protect the endometrium. Although not licensed yet in the UK for this indication, a Mirena IUS can be used to provide both contraception and endometrial protection and can be particularly useful if the woman has unacceptable progestogenic side-effects such as bloating, acne or premenstrual syndrome symptoms.[25] Changing the progestogen to dydrogesterone may also reduce progestogenic side-effects.

Switching from sequential to continuous combined therapy

When women with a uterus are postmenopausal and still require HRT for symptom control, they should be switched from sequential to continuous combined preparations; 80% of women are postmenopausal at the age of 54 years. Most women who have had six months without any bleeding (or if they have had hormonal tests and were found to have repeated raised FSH levels after the mid-40s) are postmenopausal, but the older the woman the more likely this is. You will need to discuss with Ms Mind how to switch from a sequential preparation, as she is still quite young and may have irregular bleeding if she transfers to a combined preparation at this stage. Even in older women, warn them that they may have some light irregular bleeding in the first three months but it should gradually diminish.

After discussing the advantages and disadvantages of HRT, the arrangement in clinic may be to refer patients on to the specialist nurse to continue the management or back to the GP – you will need to establish what the guidelines for the clinic suggest.

How long should HRT be continued?[26]

> **Case study 10.3**
>
> Mrs Lean has been referred from another specialist. She is a 54 year old who looks older than her years. She has had asthma all her life and still requires occasional oral steroids. She is on high-dose inhaled steroids, is small and thin and takes no exercise. She had a hysterectomy 12 years ago, after several trials of medical treatment for menorrhagia, and went on HRT shortly afterwards. She stopped HRT a year ago on the advice of her GP, but the respiratory specialist has referred her to the clinic because of her menopausal symptoms and risk of osteoporosis.

Discuss with Mrs Lean what she would prefer to do. If her menopausal symptoms are few or bearable, she may prefer to consider alternative bone-protective therapy (*see* Table 10.2). She may have symptoms that have been misattributed to the menopause. If her symptoms are clearly menopause-related, then the benefits of symptom relief and prevention of osteoporosis would probably outweigh any risks. She should have a bone-density measurement to establish a baseline from which to monitor treatment for her higher risk of osteoporosis. If she has clear menopausal symptoms, then HRT would give her relief and protect her skeleton, but a full discussion of the benefits and risks would be needed to ensure concordance.

Treatment of flushes and other symptoms

Continue while symptoms affect the quality of life, but re-evaluate benefits and risks after symptoms have resolved and have a trial without HRT.

Prevention or treatment of osteoporosis

HRT would have to be continued for life as bone mineral density falls once treatment is stopped. Most women and their health professionals will choose to transfer to other bone-protective agents (*see* Table 10.2) once menopausal symptoms have stopped.

Premature menopause

Continue until at least the median age of menopause (51 years), then re-evaluate benefits and risks. It is likely that Mrs Lean had an early menopause – hysterectomy is known to increase the risk of an early menopause. When she stopped HRT she was only 53 years old. Explain to her that, as this is only two years after the age of the average menopause, she was only at the same risk as someone who had been on HRT for two years. Her risks for continuing HRT at present are quite low, especially as she can take oestrogen without progestogens. You may want to give her some statistics about the risks of breast cancer (*see* Table 10.1).

Table 10.1: Additional breast cancers occurring over time with use of HRT[16]

	Length of HRT use		
	2 years	5 years	10 years
Oestrogen alone	0.7	2	5[a]
Combined HRT	2	8	22

[a] although the figures from the most recently published report of the Women's Health Initiative trial give no extra risk from oestrogen only HRT.[27]

Non-oestrogen treatments

After discussion about the benefits and risks of HRT you may advise against HRT, or Mrs Lean may decide against it. Other medication should then be considered if she has risk factors.

Osteoporosis

If the main indication for treatment is prevention or treatment of osteoporosis, then other medication may be preferable (*see* Table 10.2).

Table 10.2: Prevention and treatment of osteoporosis: Royal College of Physicians' grade of recommendations for therapy[7]

	Spine	Hip
Bisphosphonates:		
Etridronate	A	B
Aledronate	A	A
Risedronate	A	A
Calcium and vitamin D	ND	A
Calcium	A	B
Calcitriol	A	ND
Calcitonin	A	B
Selective oestrogen receptor modulators	A	ND

A: good evidence from randomly controlled trials.

B: evidence from observational or case-controlled trials.

ND: not demonstrated.

Selective oestrogen receptor modulators (SERMs) have been shown to have some effect on bone density. They act as oestrogens in some locations and anti-oestrogens in others. Tamoxifen, the first SERM, is widely used as a treatment for breast cancer containing oestrogen receptors. Its use is associated with a raised risk of venous thrombosis and of endometrial cancer.[24] Raloxifene, the second SERM to be commercially available, has shown a good reduction of the risk of breast cancer in people receiving it for prevention of osteoporosis. The coronary heart risk was also reduced. Further long-term studies are needed to confirm these findings. SERMs increase hot flushes and the risk of venous thrombosis. Trials are underway to determine if a combination of a low-dose oestradiol with a SERM might improve the risk profile. This would relieve hot flushes, protect the breast and bone mass and, it is hoped, have a neutral effect on the endometrium.

NICE is expected to report in June 2005 on the assessment of fracture risk and the prevention of osteoporotic fractures in individuals at high risk. The National Osteoporosis Society (NOS) has prepared a submission to NICE that gives a good summary of the current treatments available. NOS has also criticised the preliminary advice proposed by NICE, which would severely restrict treatment.[28]

Hot flushes and other symptoms[29]

Progestogens can be helpful, e.g. norethisterone 5 mg/day or megestrol acetate 40 mg/day. Clonidine has also been shown to reduce flushing but this research was based on one trial when it was used transdermally. This formulation is not currently available in the UK. Early results from trials suggest that selective serotonin reuptake inhibitors (SSRIs) e.g. venlafaxine/paroxetine may be helpful although they are not yet licensed for this indication.

Investigation of a premature menopause

Case study 10.4

Mrs Early has been referred for advice. She is 30 years old and has not had any menstrual periods for 14 months. She tells you that her mother had an early menopause and her sister, who is two years older than her, has been upset to find that she cannot have a child because of ovarian failure. Several pregnancy tests have been negative and she has had one blood test showing a raised level of FSH. She is only slightly overweight with a BMI of 27 and examination is normal with no hirsutes. She has had no illnesses or treatment such as radiotherapy or chemotherapy.

You explain to Mrs Early that an early menopause means the woman's ovaries have spontaneously stopped working before she has reached the age of 40 years. The usual criteria for diagnosis are at least four months' amenorrhoea and two FSH levels above 40 mU/ml performed at least a month apart. Women can be affected in their teens or early 20s. Some possible causes include:

- familial early menopause
- chromosomal abnormalities such as galactosaemia, congenital adrenal hyperplasia, Turner's syndrome, fragile X syndrome
- autoimmune conditions such as hypothyroidism, Crohn's disease, systemic lupus erythematosus or rheumatoid arthritis
- endocrine dysfunction such as hypothyroidism, a virilising tumour producing testosterone, a pituitary tumour suppressing ovarian function, or loss of pituitary function following delivery (Sheehan's syndrome)
- eating disorders or over-exercise conditions, e.g. in marathon runners or ballet dancers
- drug abuse
- medication such as phenothiazines
- ovarian ablation following surgery, radiotherapy or chemotherapy
- uterine obstruction (Asherman's syndrome) due to adhesions following uterine surgery
- cervical stenosis following cervical treatment such as conisation
- viral infections, such as mumps or cytomegalovirus, are thought possibly to trigger premature menopause in some women, although the association may be coincidental
- unknown causes that are labelled as idiopathic ovarian failure.

Diagnosis

You tell Mrs Early that you will try and determine why she has a premature menopause to rule out any serious complaint that might need other treatment. The investigations you arrange should include:

- FSH and oestradiol levels (on day three of the menses if any bleeding is occurring)
- prolactin
- repeat pregnancy tests as indicated by the history – this is still the most common cause of amenorrhoea and ovarian function may return in a proportion of people
- transvaginal ultrasound to:
  - exclude any obstruction to outflow
  - detect the presence of follicles
  - assess endometrial thickness and ovarian volume.

Once you have established that Mrs Early has a premature menopause, you might carry out:

- thyroid function and adrenal antibodies (in some areas ovarian antibody levels may be available)
- bone density scan
- genetic studies
- other tests indicated by the history or examination.

Treatment methods

There is no treatment available to make the ovaries start working again. Women with early menopause have a long period of postmenopausal life, which means they are at increased risk of health problems such as osteoporosis. It may be recommended that HRT be taken until Mrs Early reaches the typical age of menopause (around 51 years). Alternatively, she may prefer to take combined oral contraceptives. This would replace the oestrogen as well as giving her the reassurance that she is not pregnant.

Psychological counselling and support groups may help the woman come to terms with her experience.[30] She may have problems with her self-esteem, grief over her lost fertility, or fears about growing old before her time and her partner finding her unattractive. Sometimes the ovaries may spontaneously start working again, for reasons that are unknown. She will need to take contraceptive precautions in case this happens. Inform her that in 50% of women with premature ovarian syndrome, intermittent ovarian function may occur and in 10%, subsequent pregnancy may occur even some years after diagnosis.[31]

Treatment of urogenital symptoms

Case study 10.5

Mrs Lack is a plump 68 year old, who looks younger than her years. She looks disconcerted to see you and explains that she was expecting to see the doctor who is on sick leave. She had attended the clinic several years previously. She launches into her story with enthusiasm. She had been on oestrogen-only HRT since she was 49 years old having had a hysterectomy two years previously. She had tried stopping HRT several times with a return of terrible hot flushes. Last year she was persuaded by her GP to try stopping it again, and this time she gradually decreased the amount. She reduced the strength of her patch from

> 50 to 40 µg and then to 25 µg. Each time, she tells you, with great drama, those hot flushes returned – but not as badly as she remembered having them before. Now she has stopped altogether and she is so glad this appointment has arrived at last, because 'down below is just so sore'. If she and her husband try to make love, both of them end up sore, and she has even had a bit of bleeding. They have tried using KY jelly – but it was useless; it just 'rolled up in a ball and made things worse'. She adds 'I keep wanting to go to the loo as well and there's this nasty stinging feeling just when I finish going'. Her doctor has done some tests and there is no infection. She sits back looking at you expectantly.

After confirming that Mrs Lack has symptoms attributable to lack of oestrogen, you might discuss treatment with vaginally administered low-dose natural oestrogens, such as oestriol by cream or pessary, or oestradiol by tablet or from a ring.

You may encounter women with atrophic vaginitis when carrying out any vaginal examination in older women. This provides a perfect opportunity to raise the issue of urogenital symptoms or dyspareunia proactively, as many women will not initiate discussion of the subject themselves. Long-term treatment with local oestrogen is usually needed or symptoms may recur. With the recommended dosage regimes, no endometrial effects should occur and it is not necessary to add a progestogen, even in women who still have a uterus. However, the long-term safety of local oestrogens remains uncertain, so any vaginal bleeding should be investigated.

You might also talk to Mrs Lack about maintaining the tone in her pelvic floor muscles by carrying out pelvic floor exercises. You may find that the clinic has a supply of leaflets, or you might recommend a website.[32] If she has very lax tone, or finds the exercises too difficult, referral to a specialist physiotherapist is often very helpful.

As an adjunct to locally applied oestrogens, or if she has been put off using hormonal treatments by the recent publicity, recommend vaginal lubricants to purchase, together with discussion about why vaginal dryness is occurring, and reassurance that this does not mean that women should refrain from a regular sex life. Become familiar with the lubricants available in pharmacies, shops and on the internet.

Managing problems[26]

You might wish to join a professional organisation such as the British Menopause Society so that you keep up to date with a rapidly changing field.[33] It also provides advice about what care a specialist nurse can provide. You will probably find that most of the routine care in a menopause clinic is usually managed by an experienced specialist nurse. She may offer group sessions for education, individual support and management of those patients who do not have access to knowledgeable help in their own general practice. However, you may well be asked to advise on the following conditions that may require specialist intervention:

- *abnormal bleeding*:
  - before starting HRT: patients who have a sudden change in menstrual pattern, intermenstrual bleeding, postcoital bleeding or a postmenopausal bleed
  - while on sequential HRT: patients who have a change in the pattern of withdrawal bleed or breakthrough bleeding (BTB)
  - those taking continuous combined HRT: episodes of BTB for more than 4–6 months after starting or bleeding occurring after complete amenorrhoea
- *multiple treatment failures*: after more than three types of HRT preparations have been tried. Make a list what has been given and the problems encountered. You may be able to see a definite pattern of intolerance to types of progestogen, or identify unrealistic expectations of what hormonal treatment might achieve
- *confirmed venous thrombosis*: either personal history or in a first-degree relative under the age of 50 years, when oestrogens are likely to be contraindicated
- *premature menopause:* to determine the reason for the menopause occurring under 40 years of age
- *osteoporosis risk:* to help with the assessment for the treatment dose required and the response to treatment (refer for bone mineral density scans if available in your area)
- *previous or high risk of hormone-dependent cancer* e.g. breast, ovarian, endometrial cancer.

In addition, you will probably be asked to see patients with specific anxieties about their own medical conditions or those in close relatives. Be aware of how medical conditions may be affected by the menopause, or by HRT. For example, you may be asked if antihypertensive medication or lipid-regulating medication are affected by HRT. The *British National Formulary* gives little information, merely stating that interactions are unlikely with low-dose HRT.[34]

The British Menopause Society in collaboration with the RCOG has developed a special interest training programme covering the menopause (*see* Box 10.1).

Collecting data to demonstrate your learning, competence, performance and standards of service delivery

Example cycle of evidence 10.1

- Focus: clinical care
- Other relevant focus: working with colleagues

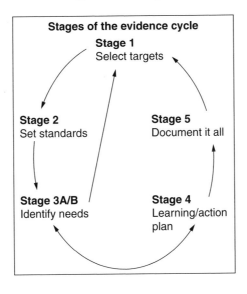

Stages of the evidence cycle

Stage 1
Select targets

Stage 2
Set standards

Stage 5
Document it all

Stage 3A/B
Identify needs

Stage 4
Learning/action plan

Case study 10.6

Mrs Muddle is 55 years old. You had arranged an ultrasound scan and a MSU was sent off when you saw her previously, as she had given a history of urinary frequency, dysuria and 'soreness down below', together with some light irregular vaginal bleeding. The appointments department had sent her another appointment for the clinic in error, as she would normally have accessed her results through her GP and only been sent an appointment if the results were abnormal. She was told at her general practice that the MSU showed no sign of infection and that the scan was normal. You ask if she still has symptoms and find that she does and has received no treatment. The labelling of the MSU as 'normal' (although it had contained many white blood cells) and her normal scan had made Mrs Muddle think that this meant she had to put up with her symptoms. You want to prevent a recurrence of this situation with other patients.

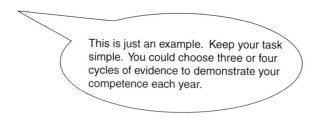

This is just an example. Keep your task simple. You could choose three or four cycles of evidence to demonstrate your competence each year.

Stage 1: Select your aspirations for good practice

The excellent doctor:

- makes an adequate assessment of the patient's condition, based on the history and, if indicated, an appropriate examination
- provides or arranges investigations or treatment where necessary
- communicates the results of investigations together with recommendations for management.

Stage 2: Set the standards for your outcomes

Outcomes might include:

- the way learning is applied
- a learnt skill
- a protocol
- a strategy that is implemented
- meeting recommended standards.

- Demonstrate consistent best practice in assessment and treatment of postmenopausal urogenital atrophy.
- Demonstrate best practice in consistency of approach through teamwork.

Stage 3A: Identify your learning needs

- Review the medical records of 10 patients who presented with urogenital symptoms, to monitor the standard of management.
- Review how results are interpreted and relayed to patients and their GPs.

Stage 3B: Identify your service needs

Any of the needs assessment exercises in 3A may also reveal service needs.

- Track what happens to reports of investigations when received.
- Discuss with other health professionals their response to MSU results that are reported as 'negative' or 'white blood cells and no growth' and what they record that the patient and the GP should be told.
- Discuss with the team what information is sent to patients and their GPs about their MSU and scan results.

Stage 4: Make and carry out a learning and action plan

- Read about urogenital atrophy, its symptoms and treatment.
- Write up the record review (that shows perhaps that most women are being treated in accordance with best practice but that a few women with urinary symptoms of urogenital atrophy are not having a recommendation or discussion of treatment options).
- Discuss the record review with other health professionals and agree to change the wording of the information about the results of the investigations to explain the options for treatment. The letter is to be copied to both the patient and the GP.
- Create a protocol for discussion with the team to highlight the best treatment options for urogenital atrophy.
- Ask the audit department to help you with including a questionnaire with the letter to the patient to conduct a small feedback study. You ask patients to return the questionnaire about their level of satisfaction with the outcome of their consultation and investigations to the audit department.

Stage 5: Document your learning, competence, performance and standards of service delivery

- Use a reminder on the audit calendar and repeat the record review in six months to confirm that the changes are working.
- Document the discussion with your team and the agreement to change the wording of the information about the results of the investigations to explain the options for treatment. You record that the letter is now copied to both the patient and the GP.
- Keep a copy of the summary of the feedback from patients who returned the satisfaction questionnaire.
- Keep a copy of the protocol you have helped to develop in your portfolio.

Case study 10.6 continued

The fail-safe mechanism for Mrs Muddle had been her appointment sent in error. You confirmed that atrophic vaginitis was the cause for her symptoms. On your recommendation, the GP prescribes local topical oestrogen therapy.

At review six months after the changes were made, you find that the team understand better the importance of communicating recommendations following negative investigations. The changes in passing on the information to patients are working well and the feedback from the questionnaire was enthusiastic. The team feel that they have become more helpful in managing patients appropriately. You and team members are more aware, and more proactive, about best practice in managing patients with urogenital atrophy.

Example cycle of evidence 10.2

- Focus: maintaining good medical practice
- Other relevant foci: working with colleagues; relationships with patients

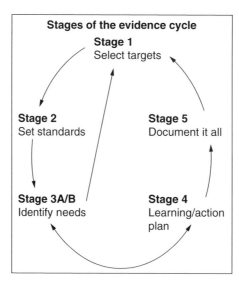

Stages of the evidence cycle

Stage 1
Select targets

Stage 2
Set standards

Stage 5
Document it all

Stage 3A/B
Identify needs

Stage 4
Learning/action plan

Case study 10.7

Mrs Manager is 56 years old. She has been taking a sequential hormone pack for seven years and attends for a routine review at the menopause clinic. She has missed or rearranged several appointments and has not been reviewed for over two years, although she has been obtaining HRT from her GP, telling him that she attends the menopause clinic. She is happy with her treatment and wishes to continue. However, she has had irregular bleeding and is annoyed when the nurse tells her that this means she will have to see the doctor. She explains impatiently that she often manipulates the timing of her bleed, as it is more convenient to do that in her busy life. She tells you that she sees no point in having a specialist nurse clinic if the nurse has to send patients back to the doctor.

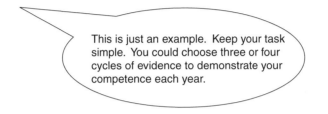

This is just an example. Keep your task simple. You could choose three or four cycles of evidence to demonstrate your competence each year.

Stage 1: Select your aspirations for good practice

The excellent doctor:

- keeps his or her knowledge and skills up to date throughout their working life, through continuing educational activities that maintain and develop competence and performance
- works with colleagues to monitor and maintain the quality of care provided
- takes part in regular and systematic clinical audit and makes improvements accordingly.

Stage 2: Set the standards for your outcomes

Outcomes might include:

- the way learning is applied
- a learnt skill
- a protocol
- a strategy that is implemented
- meeting recommended standards.

- Demonstrate best practice in management of the menopause.
- Ensure that there is a system in place for notifying GPs and patients when patient review is overdue.

Stage 3A: Identify your learning needs

- Compare your management with best current management in the provision of HRT and recommended length of treatment.
- Review the nature and quality of patient education materials including the availability of literature.

Stage 3B: Identify your service needs

> Any of the needs assessment exercises in 3A may also reveal service needs.

- Audit the use of sequential HRT in the clinic including setting standards. For example you might agree that 100% of women continuing on HRT should have had a discussion about transferring to continuous combined therapy between the ages of 52 and 55 years and 100% of those being reviewed after the age of 52 years should have had a discussion to determine if treatment is still required.
- Discuss with relevant staff the guidelines for the use of HRT.
- Track what happens to patients who have failed to attend or postponed their appointments for review.

Stage 4: Make and carry out a learning and action plan

- Perform a literature search for recent recommendations, especially any systematic reviews, for current best practice on HRT.
- Obtain guidelines for running a menopause clinic from an authoritative source, e.g. the British Menopause Society.[33]
- Discuss with colleagues how they notify patients and their GPs of the requirement for review of ongoing medication.
- Ask patients at the clinic to read and comment on a pilot letter that you might send out if they postpone or default from follow-up. Modify the letter and arrange for it to be sent automatically to the patient, with a copy to the GP, when the patient does not attend for review on the due date.

Stage 5: Document your learning, competence, performance and standards of service delivery

- Incorporate and disseminate new information in the guidelines for the menopause clinic.
- Re-audit the use of sequential HRT to confirm that the changes agreed are being implemented.

- Keep a copy of the letter and the new arrangements for sending it to patients and their GPs when they default from review.

Case study 10.7 continued

You tell Mrs Manager that a trial without her HRT treatment is recommended to establish whether she still has symptoms that require treatment and if she has irregular bleeding when not taking the HRT (as that would require investigation). You advise her that she can transfer to a continuous combined preparation if she still requires HRT. She is displeased with the change to her routine. You give her a list of websites and patient information leaflets that will further explain the rationale behind this recommendation.

    You and the specialist nurse discuss Mrs Manager's future care and decide on a joint policy to maintain a consistent approach. You feel that you are in more control of managing the risks of unsupervised long-term treatment and that patients on sequential treatment will have the opportunity to discuss discontinuing HRT or transferring to combined therapy.

Example cycle of evidence 10.3

- Focus: relationships with patients
- Other relevant focus: working with colleagues

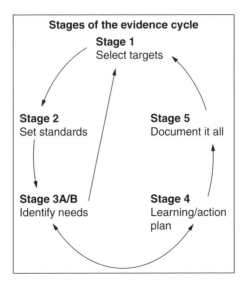

Case study 10.7 continued

When Mrs Manager returns, she is adamant she must continue on HRT as her symptoms are affecting her work. She asks angrily why she was not informed about these changes to management or the availability of patient literature before now. You tell her that patient care is continually improving and adapting to ensure that patients have the opportunity to become experts in their own care. You apologise for the fact that she had not received this information on her previous attendance.

You discuss Mrs Manager with the nurse in the clinic. Both of you feel that the patient–nurse or patient–doctor interactions with this assertive woman, who is always in a hurry, have affected the quality of care that she had received. You arrange for the same sources of patient information to be available in the consulting rooms of both doctors and nurses, and ask the nurse and reception clerk to restock this when supplies become low.

> This is just an example. Keep your task simple. You could choose three or four cycles of evidence to demonstrate your competence each year.

Stage 1: Select your aspirations for good practice

The excellent doctor:

- empowers patients to take informed decisions about their management
- apologises appropriately when things go wrong, and has an adequate complaint procedure in place.

Stage 2: Set the standards for your outcomes

Outcomes might include:

- the way learning is applied
- a learnt skill
- a protocol
- a strategy that is implemented
- meeting recommended standards.

- Demonstrate consistent best practice in patient relationships.
- Demonstrate that you recognise when your management has not gone as well as it should, apologise appropriately to the patient and take steps to remedy the deficiency.

Stage 3A: Identify your learning needs

- Record in your reflective diary types of doctor–patient interaction that create barriers to best management, from feedback from patients.
- Reflect on your skills and attitudes when consulting with authoritative or manipulative patients.

Stage 3B: Identify your service needs

Any of the needs assessment exercises in 3A may also reveal service needs.

- Enable colleagues, and staff for whom you are responsible, to recognise and attempt to remove the barriers to best management.
- Undertake a 360° survey within the team, enquiring particularly about colleagues' perceived relationships with patients.

Stage 4: Make and carry out a learning and action plan

- Ask a colleague who has done assertiveness training to facilitate role-play scenarios of difficult patient–staff interactions. The scenarios are to include those where the patient is very authoritative, resulting in the staff member behaving in a subservient or resentful manner.
- Learn how to use that recognition of doctor–patient interaction to modify your consultation style appropriately.
- Use reflective writing with an established reflective model to analyse your interactions with other authoritative patients and record your conclusions about your improvement.[35]

Stage 5: Document your learning, competence, performance and standards of service delivery

- Include your reflections and analysis within your portfolio.
- Keep records of patient and 360° surveys and subsequent planned changes.

Case study 10.7 continued

You feel that you have identified and learnt how to improve your management of powerful patients who want rapid consultations and high levels of information. You develop a much better rapport with Mrs Manager as you review her health needs and recognise that she has learnt to appear busy in order not to be challenged.

Example cycle of evidence 10.4

- Focus: working with colleagues
- Other relevant focus: teaching and training

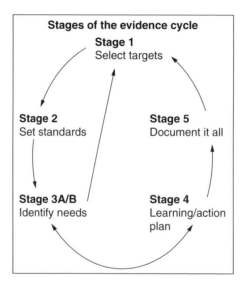

Stages of the evidence cycle

Stage 1
Select targets

Stage 2
Set standards

Stage 5
Document it all

Stage 3A/B
Identify needs

Stage 4
Learning/action plan

Case study 10.8

A PCO in your area asks if you will help to set up and run menopause clinics as they are committed to improving and widening the provision of sexual health services in the community.

This is just an example. Keep your task simple. You could choose three or four cycles of evidence to demonstrate your competence each year.

Stage 1: Select your aspirations for good practice

The excellent doctor in relationships with colleagues:

- is supportive to others undertaking a similar role
- recognises the need to share clinical expertise.

And in teaching and training:

- contributes to the education of students or colleagues willingly
- develops the skills, attitudes and practices of a competent teacher if he/she has responsibilities for teaching
- employs the principles of giving accurate feedback to enhance the performance of others.

Stage 2: Set the standards for your outcomes

Outcomes might include:

- the way learning is applied
- a learnt skill
- a protocol
- a strategy that is implemented
- meeting recommended standards.

- Demonstrate and communicate consistent best practice in providing clinical care for menopausal problems.
- Demonstrate and communicate consistent best practice in providing services for patients who require advice and treatment for menopausal problems.

Stage 3A: Identify your learning needs

- Review the feedback you have received from students on courses, workshops and individual learning sessions that you have run in the last 12 months and reflect on any learning needs revealed.
- Ask for peer review for the course material you have written for training.
- Check by comparing against guidelines that the knowledge and skills you are imparting are up to date and best practice.

Stage 3B: Identify your service needs

Any of the needs assessment exercises in 3A may also reveal service needs.

- Find out what additional help will be available to these doctors and nurses with a special interest and how the PCO intends to help them develop new clinical skills.
- Discuss how the dual demands of service provision and education and training needs can be effectively accommodated.
- Establish a group of interested health professionals with expertise in the menopause who can help take this initiative forward, rather than attempting to carry the load alone.

Stage 4: Make and carry out a learning and action plan

- Undertake a refresher teaching and assessing course to ensure an optimal approach to students and junior staff.
- Approach the medical and nursing departments within the local university to see if they would consider developing accredited courses on managing the menopause.
- Write, and obtain feedback on, training materials for the topic.
- Read widely about the subject of the menopause, both the literature for health professionals and for patients.
- Arrange for the PwSIs to attend your clinic as observers. This will help you to establish what their learning needs might be.

Stage 5: Document your learning, competence, performance and standards of service delivery

- Record the feedback from PwSIs who attend your menopause clinic as observers.
- Log the feedback on your teaching, training and written materials.

- Record your reflections on what changes you need to make after attending the refresher course on training and assessment.

Case study 10.8 continued

You establish an expert advisory group where everyone agrees to contribute to the education of PwSIs who are interested in running menopause clinics. The university is more than happy to develop a course with the help of local clinicians and plans to include a variety of educational processes including seminars and clinical placement opportunities, and to use a problem-based learning approach to encourage analysis of case histories.

References

1   www.rcog.org.uk/mainpages.asp?PageID=1042

2   Bungay GT, Vessey MP and McPherson CK (1980) Study of symptoms in middle life with special reference to the menopause. *British Medical Journal.* **281:** 181–3.

3   Nugent D and Balen A (1999) Pregnancy in the older woman. *Journal of the British Menopause Society.* **5:** 132–4.

4   Brechin S and Gebbie A (1999) *Perimenopausal Contraception: FACT review.* www.ffprhc.org.uk

5   Hunter MS (1996) Depression and menopause. *British Medical Journal.* **313:** 1217–18.

6   Nicol-Smith L (1996) Causality, menopause, and depression: a critical review of the literature. *British Medical Journal.* **313:** 1229–32.

7   Anonymous (1999) *Osteoporosis. Clinical guidelines for prevention and treatment.* Royal College of Physicians, London.

8   Black DM, Steinbuch M, Palermo L *et al.* (2001) An assessment tool for predicting fracture risk in postmenopausal women. *Osteoporosis International.* **12:** 519–28.

9   Guthrie JR (1999) Role of lifestyle approaches in the management of the menopause. *Journal of the British Menopause Society.* **5:** 25–8.

10   Ernst E (1999) Herbal remedies as a treatment of some frequent symptoms during menopause. *Journal of the British Menopause Society.* **5:** 117–20.

11   Davis SR (2001) Phytoestrogen therapy for menopausal symptoms? *British Medical Journal.* **323:** 354–5.

12   www.acupuncture.org.uk/content/Library/menopause_bp5.pdf

13   Bandolier (October 1998) Alternatives for the menopause. *Bandolier.* **56-3.** www.jr2.ox.ac.uk/bandolier/band56/b56-3.html

14   Rees M, Purdie D and Hope S (2003) *The Menopause. What you need to know.* BMS Publications, Marlow. www.the-bms.org

15   Menopause Matters website. www.menopausematters.co.uk

16   Committee on Safety of Medicines (2003) HRT: update on the risk of breast cancer and long-term safety. *Current Problems in Pharmocovigilance.* **29:** 1–3. www.mca.gov.uk

17   Pitkin J, Rees MCP, Gray S *et al.* (2003) Managing the menopause. British Menopause Society Council Consensus statement on hormone replacement therapy. *Journal of the British Menopause Society.* **9:** 129–31.

18   Panay N (2004) Hormone replacement therapy: the way forward. *Journal of Family Planning and Reproductive Health Care.* **30:** 21–3.

19   Rymer J, Wilson R and Ballard K (2003) Making decisions about hormone replacement therapy. *British Medical Journal.* **326:** 322–6.

20   Collaborative group on Hormonal Factors in Breast Cancer (1997) Breast cancer and hormone replacement therapy: collaborative reanalysis of data from 51 epidemiological studies of 52 705 women with breast cancer and 108 411 women without breast cancer. *Lancet.* **350:** 1047–59.

21   Writing Group for the Women's Health Initiative Investigators (2002) Risks and benefits of estrogen plus progestin in healthy postmenopausal women: principal results from the Women's Health Initiative randomized controlled trial. *Journal of the American Medical Association.* **288:** 321–33.

22   Million Women Study Collaborators (2003) Breast cancer and hormone replacement therapy in the Million Women Study. *Lancet.* **362:** 419–27.

23   Buckler HM, Kalsi PK, Cantrill JA and Anderson DC (1995) An audit of oestradiol levels and implant frequency in women undergoing subcutaneous implant therapy. *Clinical Endocrinology (Oxford).* **42:** 445–50.

24   Davis SR (2003) Menopause: new therapies. *Menopause Journal of Australia.* **178:** 634–7. Full text available with references on www.mja.com.au

25   Raudaskoski T, Tapanainen J, Tomas E *et al.* (2002) Intrauterine 10 microgram and 20 microgram levonorgestrel systems in postmenopausal women receiving oral oestrogen therapy: clinical endometrial and metabolic response. *British Journal of Obstetrics and Gynaecology.* **109:** 135–44.

26   Rees M and Purdie DW (eds) (2002) *Management of the Menopause* (3e). The British Menopause Society, Marlow.

27   The Women's Health Initiative Steering Committee (2004) Effects of conjugated equine estrogen in post menopausal women with hysterectomy. The Women's Health Initiative randomized controlled trial. *Journal of the American Medical Association.* **291:** 1701–12.

28   www.nos.org.uk/PDF/nice_submission.pdf

29   Morris E and Rymer J (2003) Menopausal symptoms. *Clinical Evidence Concise.* **10:** 398–9. www.clinicalevidence.com

30   Premature Ovarian Failure Support Group (POFSG) website. www.pofsupport. org

31   Conway G, Kaltas G, Patel A *et al.* (1996) Characterisation of idiopathic premature ovarian failure. *Fertility and Sterility.* **65**: 337–41.

32   Continence Foundation website, pelvic floor exercises for women. www. continence-foundation.org.uk/symptoms-and-treatments/pelvic-floor-exercises. php

33   British Menopause Society website. www.the-bms.org

34   Joint Formulary Committee (2004) *British National Formulary.* British Medical Association and Royal Pharmaceutical Society of Great Britain, London. www. bnf.org

35   Schön, D (1983) *The Reflective Practitioner: How professionals think in action.* Basic Books, New York.

And finally

We hope that you have found that the stages in our 'cycle of evidence' are a useful approach to gathering information about what you need to learn. You can also use it to identify improvements you or others need to make to the way you deliver services.

It is easy to feel overwhelmed by the magnitude of the task to demonstrate that you are competent and perform consistently well as a doctor, in order to retain your licence to practise. Remember that you should be producing evidence about the breadth of your practice every five years. Take your time and select three or four cycles of evidence each year, that span several headings of *Good Medical Practice* at one time.[1]

Ask others for help. Your district tutor, clinical director and secretary should be able to help you to collect information about what you need to learn, or about gaps in services. You can delegate much of the administrative side. Your colleagues or your patients will be well placed to help you to set your aspirations for good practice and set achievable standards for your outcomes – of learning and improvements in service delivery. Perhaps your CPD tutor can help you to develop learning and action in your PDP. These cycles of evidence will be the nucleus of your PDP. Colleagues in the team can support you in documenting the evidence of your competence, performance and subsequent standards of service delivery. Other books in this series might help you to look at specific clinical areas, especially those where quality frameworks or special interests require your attention. Remember to visit this book's supporting website, which includes useful website links.[2]

So the evidence will be there ready to submit for appraisal interviews or revalidation, but the results will show what a good doctor you really are. This should give you increasing confidence and self-respect. Enjoy your professional glow.

References

1 General Medical Council (2001) *Good Medical Practice.* General Medical Council, London.

2 http://repromed.mattersonline.net

Index